Renal and Urinary Systems

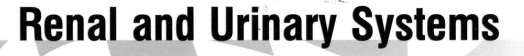

First and second edition authors:

Nisha Mirpuri

Pratiksha Patel

Shreelata Data

Third edition authors:

Robert Thomas

Bethany Stanley

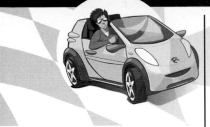

4th Edition

CRASH COURSE

SERIES EDITOR:

Dan Horton-Szar

BSc(Hons) MBBS(Hons) MRCGP
Northgate Medical Practice
Canterbury, Kent, UK

FACULTY ADVISOR:

Kevin Harris

Medical Director and Honorary Consultant Nephrologist
University Hospitals of Leicester NHS Trust, Leicester, UK
Reader in the Department of Infection, Immunity and Inflammation
University of Leicester, Leicester, UK

Renal and Urinary Systems

Timothy Jones

MBChB(Hons)
Medical Student, University of Leicester Medical School,
Leicester, UK

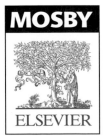

MOSBY

ELSEVIER

Edinburgh London New York Oxford Philadelphia St Louis Sydney Toronto 2015

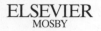

ELSEVIER
MOSBY

Commissioning Editor: Jeremy Bowes
Development Editor: Carole McMurray
Project Manager: Andrew Riley
Designer: Stewart Larking
Icon Illustrations: Geo Parkin
Illustration Manager: Jennifer Rose
Illustrator: Cactus

First edition 1998

Second edition 2003

Third edition 2007

Fourth edition 2012

Updated Fourth edition 2015

ISBN: 978-0-7234-3859-5

British Library Cataloguing in Publication Data
A catalogue record for this book is available from the British Library

Library of Congress Cataloging in Publication Data
A catalog record for this book is available from the Library of Congress

Notices
Knowledge and best practice in this field are constantly changing. As new research and experience broaden our understanding, changes in research methods, professional practices, or medical treatment may become necessary.

Practitioners and researchers must always rely on their own experience and knowledge in evaluating and using any information, methods, compounds, or experiments described herein. In using such information or methods they should be mindful of their own safety and the safety of others, including parties for whom they have a professional responsibility.

With respect to any drug or pharmaceutical products identified, readers are advised to check the most current information provided (i) on procedures featured or (ii) by the manufacturer of each product to be administered, to verify the recommended dose or formula, the method and duration of administration, and contraindications. It is the responsibility of practitioners, relying on their own experience and knowledge of their patients, to make diagnoses, to determine dosages and the best treatment for each individual patient, and to take all appropriate safety precautions.

To the fullest extent of the law, neither the Publisher nor the authors, contributors, or editors, assume any liability for any injury and/or damage to persons or property as a matter of products liability, negligence or otherwise, or from any use or operation of any methods, products, instructions, or ideas contained in the material herein.

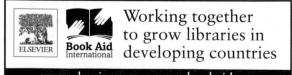
Printed in China

Last digit is the print line: 10 9 8 7 6 5 4 3 2 1

Series editor foreword

The *Crash Course* series was first published in 1997 and now, 15 years on, we are still going strong. Medicine never stands still, and the work of keeping this series relevant for today's students is an ongoing process. These fourth editions build on the success of the previous titles and incorporate new and revised material, to keep the series up-to-date with current guidelines for best practice, and recent developments in medical research and pharmacology.

We always listen to feedback from our readers, through focus groups and student reviews of the *Crash Course* titles. For the fourth editions we have completely re-written our self-assessment material to keep up with today's single-best answer and extended matching question formats. The artwork and layout of the titles has also been largely re-worked to make it easier on the eye during long sessions of revision.

Despite fully revising the books with each edition, we hold fast to the principles on which we first developed the series. *Crash Course* will always bring you all the information you need to revise in compact, manageable volumes that integrate basic medical science and clinical practice. The books still maintain the balance between clarity and conciseness, and provide sufficient depth for those aiming at distinction. The authors are medical students and junior doctors who have recent experience of the exams you are now facing, and the accuracy of the material is checked by a team of faculty advisors from across the UK.

I wish you all the best for your future careers!

Dr Dan Horton-Szar

Series Editor

Prefaces

Author preface

This book was written with the aim of presenting subjects that are complex and important for medical students in a concise and understandable way. It follows the successful approach of previous editions, being written by medical students thus pitched at an appropriate level for my busy peers.

For the new edition the content has been reorganised to remove the separation between clinical and pre-clinical subjects. Thus, one will now read about the physiology of osmolality control alongside hyponatraemia and hypernatraemia. This has removed an element of repetition in the text and immediately highlights the relevance of the basic medical science.

The self assessment section now consists of single best answer and extended matching questions to reflect the trend of examination at medical school and beyond. I hope that you find the book useful and interesting and that you enjoy using it for learning and revision.

Tim Jones

Faculty advisor

Diseases of the urinary tract have traditionally been seen as a challenging subject for medical students. This *Crash Course* book sets out to ensure the subject matter is presented in a logical and concise way making the subject matter readily accessible to the student. As with all *Crash Course* books, the text is authored by a medical student with expert input from a Faculty Advisor – me – and the series editor.

This 4th edition of this *Crash Course: Renal and Urinary Systems* book has undergone extensive revision. The text has been reorganised to ensure that there is integration between 'preclinical' pathophysiological concepts and 'clinical' presentations of disease. This approach will provide the student with a logical theoretical basis for solving the sorts of problems that are commonly encountered in clinical practice. At the same time the text has been updated with reference to the latest internationally recognized classifications of both chronic kidney disease (CKD) and acute kidney injury (AKI).

A revised self assessment section is designed to provide the student with a basis on which to ensure they have a well grounded understanding of the subject matter – not only to ensure they a ready for their exams but also to stimulate them to continue with self-directed learning.

Kevin Harris

Acknowledgements

I am very grateful to Dr Kevin Harris for his help and advice throughout the project. Thank you also to the staff at Elsevier, particularly Carole McMurray for the encouragement in the production of this edition.

Figure credits

Figures 2.2, 2.6 and 5.5 from Koeppen BM, Stanton B 1996 Renal physiology, 2nd edn. Mosby Year Book

Figure 3.21 Berne RM, LevyMN 1996 Physiology, 3rd edn. Mosby Year Book

Figure 7.7 adapted from O'Callaghan, The Kidney at a glance 2001 Blackwell science.

Figure 8.27 redrawn with permission from L Impey, Obstetrics and gynaecology 1999.

Figures 8.16, 8.20, 8.22 and 8.29 from Williams G, Mallick NP 1994 Color atlas of renal diseases, 2nd edn. Mosby Year Book

Figures 8.23 and 8.28 from Lloyd-Davis RW et al 1994 Color atlas of urology, 2nd edn. Mosby Year Book.

Figure 8.30 from Johnson RJ, Feehally J 2000 Comprehensive nephrology. Mosby Year Book.

Thanks to Dr D Rickards, Dr TO Nunan and Mr RS Cole for clinical images.

Contents

Organization of the kidneys ①

OVERVIEW OF THE KIDNEY AND URINARY TRACT

The kidneys lie in the retroperitoneum on the posterior abdominal wall on either side of the vertebral column (T11–L3). The right kidney is displaced by the liver, so it is 12 mm lower than the left kidney. The adult kidney is approximately 11 cm long and 6 cm wide, with a mass of 140 g. Each kidney is composed of two main regions:

• An outer dark brown cortex
• An inner pale medulla and renal pelvis.

The renal pelvis contains the major renal blood vessels and the origins of the ureter. Each kidney consists of 1 million nephrons, which span the cortex and medulla and are bound together by connective tissue containing blood vessels, nerves and lymphatics.

The kidneys form the upper part of the urinary tract. The urine produced by the kidneys is transported to the bladder by two ureters. The lower urinary tract consists of the bladder and the urethra.

Clinical Note

Approximately 1–1.5 L of urine is produced by the kidneys each day – the volume and osmolality vary according to fluid intake and fluid loss.

The urinary tract epithelium is impermeable to water and solutes unlike the nephrons in the kidney, so the composition of urine is not altered as it is transported to the bladder. The bladder contents are emptied via the urethra, expulsion from the body being controlled by an external sphincter. Both the upper and the lower urinary tracts are innervated by the autonomic nervous system.

Figure 1.1 shows the anatomy of the kidneys and urinary tract.

Functions of the kidney and the urinary tract

1. **Excretion**: of waste products and drugs – this involves selective reabsorption and excretion of substances as they pass through the nephron
2. **Regulation**: of body fluid volume and ionic composition. The kidneys have a major role in homeostasis (the maintenance of a constant internal environment) and are also involved in maintaining the acid–base balance
3. **Endocrine**: the kidneys are involved in the synthesis of renin (which generates angiotensin I from angiotensinogen, and thus has a role in blood pressure and sodium balance), erythropoietin (which controls erythrocyte production) and prostaglandins (involved in regulation of renal function)
4. **Metabolism**: Vitamin D is metabolized to its active form. The kidney is a major site for the catabolism of low-molecular-weight proteins including several hormones such as insulin, parathyroid hormone and calcitonin.

Fig. 1.1 Anatomy of the posterior abdominal wall showing the renal and urinary system. 1, liver; 2, stomach; 3, second part of the duodenum; 4, pancreas.

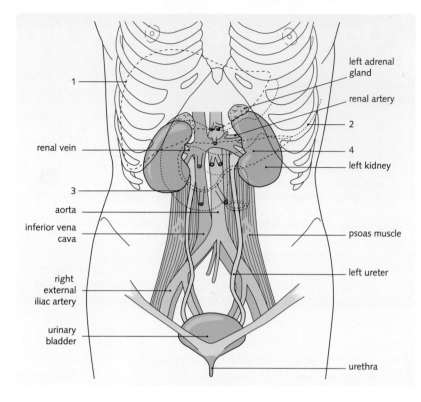

GENERAL ORGANIZATION OF THE KIDNEYS

Macroscopic organization

The kidneys lie in a fatty cushion (perinephric fat) contained within the renal fascia. They have three capsular layers:

1. Fascial (renal fascia)
2. Fatty (perinephric fascia)
3. True (fibrous capsule).

The anatomical relations of the kidneys are as follows:

- **Anterior** (Fig. 1.2): to the right kidney – liver, second part of the duodenum and the colon; to the left kidney – stomach, pancreas, spleen, jejunum and descending colon
- **Posterior**: diaphragm, quadratus lumborum, psoas, 12th rib and three nerves (subcostal, iliohypogastric and ilioinguinal)
- **Medial**: hilum (a deep fissure containing the renal vessels, nerves, lymphatics and the renal pelvis); to the left kidney – aorta; to the right kidney – inferior vena cava
- **Superior**: adrenal gland.

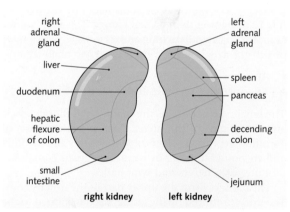

Fig. 1.2 Anterior relations of the right and left kidneys.

Within the kidney, the ureter continues as the renal pelvis, which lies in a deep fissure called the hilum. The outer border of the renal pelvis divides into two or three major divisions (calyces). These subdivide into a number of minor calyces and are each indented by a papilla of renal tissue called the renal pyramid. It is here that the collecting tubules empty the urine. Along with the renal pelvis, the renal artery, vein, nerve and lymphatics all enter the medial border of the kidney at the hilum (Fig. 1.3).

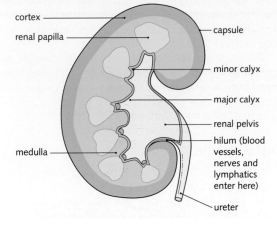

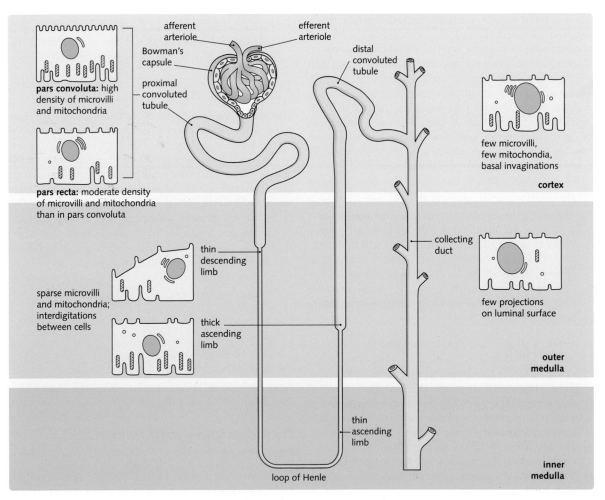

Fig. 1.3 Longitudinal section showing the macroscopic organization of the kidney.

The kidney is divided into two main layers:

1. Outer renal cortex (dark)
2. Inner renal medulla (paler).

The nephron and histology

Each kidney has approximately 1 million nephrons. The nephron (Fig. 1.4) is the functional unit of the kidney and consists of:

- A renal corpuscle (Bowman's capsule and the glomerulus)
- Tubule (proximal tubule, loop of Henle, distal tubule and collecting duct).

There are two types of nephron, depending on the length of the loop of Henle:

- **Cortical nephrons**: these have renal corpuscles in the outer part of the cortex, with a correspondingly short loop of Henle

Fig. 1.4 The structure of a nephron and the main histological features of the different cell types within it.

- **Juxtamedullary nephrons**: these have larger renal corpuscles in the inner third of the cortex, with long loops of Henle extending into the medulla.

In the human kidney, 85% of the nephrons are cortical nephrons and the remaining 15% are juxtamedullary nephrons.

Glomerulus

The glomerulus is formed by the invagination of a ball of capillaries into the Bowman's capsule, which is the blind end of a nephron. It has a diameter of approximately 200 μm.

The function of the glomerulus is to produce a protein-free filtrate from the blood in the glomerular capillaries. The capillaries are supplied by the afferent arterioles and drained by the efferent arterioles. The filtration membrane of the renal corpuscle is made up of three layers and is fundamental to kidney function.

Proximal tubule

The proximal tubule continues from the renal corpuscle. It is 15 mm long and 55 μm in diameter. Its wall is composed of a single layer of cuboidal cells, which interdigitate extensively and are connected by tight junctions at their luminal surfaces. The luminal edge of each cell is made up of millions of microvilli, forming a dense brush border that increases the surface area available for absorption of tubular filtrate. At the base of each cell there are infoldings of the cell membrane (see Fig. 1.4). The extracellular space between the cells is known as the lateral intercellular space.

The structure of the proximal tubule varies along its length:

- The first part is convoluted (pars convoluta) and cells have an increased density of microvilli and a greater number of mitochondria than cells in the second straight part. This suggests a role in transport of substances across the lumen and the filtrate
- The second straight part (pars recta) leads on to the first part of the loop of Henle (the thin descending limb).

Loop of Henle

The loop of Henle consists of a single layer of flattened squamous cells, which form a thin-walled, hairpin-shaped tube. The cells of the thin descending segment interdigitate sparingly and have few mitochondria and microvilli on the luminal surface (see Fig. 1.4). This segment ends at the tip of the hairpin loop.

The thin ascending segment is 2 mm long and 20 μm in diameter. Its structure is similar to the preceding part of the tubule (the pars recta), except that the cells have extensive interdigitations. This might have a role in the

active transport and permeability properties of the cells. There is an abrupt transition between the thin and thick ascending segments and the level of this depends on the length of the loop.

The thick ascending segment is 12 mm in length and consists of a single layer of columnar cells. The luminal membrane is invaginated to form many projections, although there is no brush border and there are few infoldings of the basal membrane.

Distal tubule

The distal convoluted tubule is the continuation of the loop of Henle into the cortex, ending in the collecting ducts. The cells have very few microvilli, no brush border and basal infoldings surrounding mitochondria that gradually decrease towards the collecting ducts (see Fig. 1.4). The basal membranes have Na^+/K^+ ATPase pump activity (see p. 27).

Different cell types in this part of the tubule include:

- **Principal cells (P cells)**: these contain few mitochondria and respond to antidiuretic hormone (ADH) – also known as vasopressin
- **Intercalated cells (I cells)**: these contain lots of mitochondria and secrete hydrogen ions (H^+).

Collecting ducts

The cortical collecting ducts are 20 mm long. They are lined with cuboidal cells that have a few projections on the luminal surface (see Fig. 1.4).

The ducts pass through the renal cortex and medulla and, at the apices of the renal pyramids, drain the urine into the renal pelvis. The renal pelvis is lined by transitional epithelium.

In the cortex each collecting duct drains approximately six distal tubules. In the medulla the collecting ducts join together in pairs to form ducts of Bellini and from here drain into the renal calyx.

> **HINTS AND TIPS**
>
> Renal function and urine formation depends on three basic processes:
> 1. Glomerular filtration
> 2. Tubular reabsorption
> 3. Tubular secretion.

Blood supply and vascular structure

The kidneys receive 20–25% of the total cardiac output (1.2 L/min) via the right and left renal arteries, which branch directly off the abdominal aorta at the level L1.

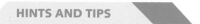

The right renal artery is longer than the left as it passes posterior to the vena cava. They branch to form interlobar arteries, which further divide to form the arcuate arteries (located at the junction between the cortex and medulla). The interlobular arteries arise at 90° to the arcuate arteries through the cortex, dividing to form the afferent arterioles. These form glomerular capillary networks (Fig. 1.5) and come together to form the efferent arterioles.

The efferent arterioles drain blood from the glomerular capillaries and act as portal vessels (i.e. carry blood from one capillary network to another).

- In the outer two-thirds of the cortex the efferent arterioles form a network of peritubular capillaries that supplies all cortical parts of the nephron
- In the inner third of the cortex the efferent arterioles follow a hairpin course to form a capillary network surrounding the loops of Henle and the collecting ducts down into the medulla. These vessels are known as the vasa recta.

The vasa recta and the peritubular capillaries drain into the left and right renal veins. These lie anterior to the renal arteries and drain directly into the inferior vena cava.

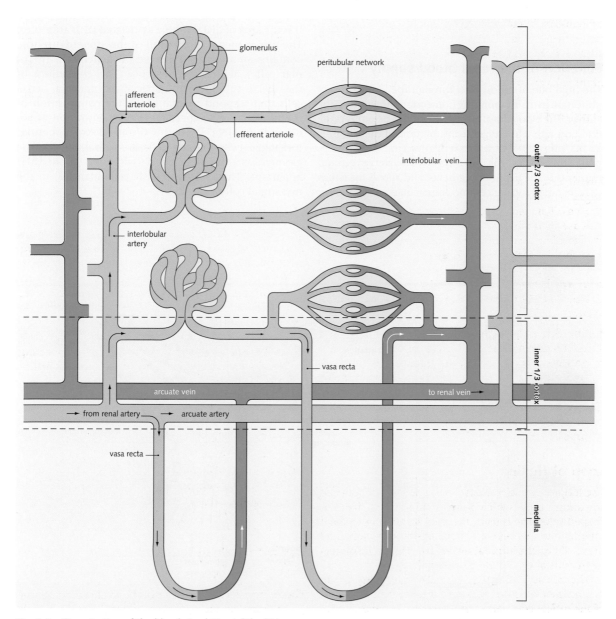

Fig. 1.5 Organization of the blood circulation of the kidney.

The left renal vein is three times longer than the right as it passes anterior to the abdominal aorta.

Clinical Note

The intricate structure and complex nature of the renal blood supply make it very susceptible to damage. The glomerulus may be damaged by high blood pressure and high blood sugar levels in diabetes mellitus. Inflammatory conditions such as glomerulonephritis also lead to disruption of the glomerular capillary filter which results in the presence of blood and protein in the urine (haematuria and proteinuria, respectively).

Function of the renal blood supply

The high rate of blood flow through the kidney is very important in maintaining the homeostatic functions of the kidney. The blood flow through the kidney determines the filtration rate. The oxygen consumption of the kidney is 18 mL/min – 50% of which is involved in Na^+ reabsorption in the tubules. The vasa recta helps deliver oxygen and nutrients to the nephron segments, and allows the return of reabsorbed substances into the circulation.

Although there is substantial blood flow, the arteriovenous oxygen difference is only about 15 mL/L, compared with 62 mL/L in the brain and 114 mL/L in the heart. This means that the oxygen extraction in the kidney is not as efficient as in other organs as a result of shunting of blood in the vasa recta through its hairpin structure.

Juxtaglomerular apparatus

The juxtaglomerular apparatus (JGA) (Fig. 1.6) is located where the thick ascending loop of Henle passes back up into the cortex and lies adjacent to the renal corpuscle and arterioles of its own nephron. It is the area of distal tubule associated with arterioles. The tunica media in the wall of the afferent arteriole contains an area of specialized thickened cells (granular cells), which secrete renin. The epithelium of the distal tubule forms specialized macula densa cells that respond to changes in the composition of the tubular fluid, especially the concentration of sodium ions ($[Na^+]$) in the filtrate. Extraglomerular mesangial cells or lacis cells are found outside the glomerulus, in association with the glomerular apparatus. They are contractile cells identical to the mesangial cells.

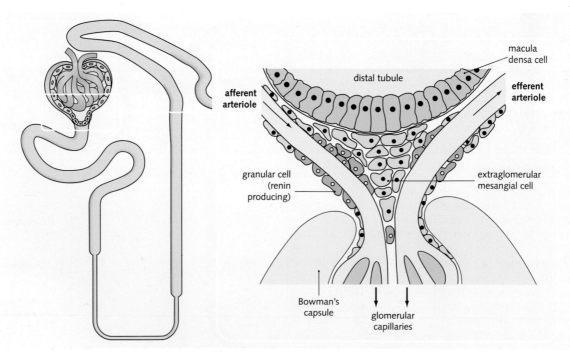

Fig. 1.6 Histology of the juxtaglomerular apparatus.

Hormones produced by the kidney

Renin

Renin is a protein that acts on angiotensinogen to form angiotensin I, which in turn is converted to angiotensin II. Angiotensin II is a potent vasoconstrictor affecting blood pressure, tubular reabsorption of Na^+, and aldosterone secretion from the adrenal glands. Renin release is stimulated by sympathetic stimulation of the granular cells or a decrease in filtrate Na^+ concentration. The latter can occur following a fall in plasma volume, vasodilation of the afferent arterioles and renal ischaemia.

Erythropoietin

The kidney is the major source (85%) of erythropoietin (EPO) production in the adult; in fetal life the liver also produces EPO. It is produced by the peritubular interstitium and the cells of the inner cortex. EPO-sensitive cells are the erythrocyte stem cells found in the bone marrow and the effect of the hormone is to increase the production of erythrocytes, resulting in an increase in the oxygen-carrying capacity of the blood. The half-life of EPO is 5 h.

Clinical use of EPO

Hypoxia, anaemia and renal ischaemia all stimulate EPO synthesis (this is a prostaglandin-mediated response). Increased secretion can be seen in polycystic kidney disease and renal cell carcinoma, resulting in polycythaemia. Patients with advanced CKD (typically stage 4) often have inappropriately low EPO secretion, resulting in normochromic normocytic anaemia. Administration of recombinant EPO (either intravenous or subcutaneous) will correct the anaemia of CKD.

Vitamin D

Vitamin D is a steroid hormone that is found in foods and is also synthesized in the skin from 7-dehydrocholesterol in the presence of sunlight. This naturally occurring vitamin D (cholecalciferol) is hydroxylated in the liver to form 25-hydroxy-cholecalciferol ($25(OH)D_3$). It is further hydroxylated in the proximal tubules under the influence of the enzyme 1a-hydroxylase to form the active metabolite 1,25-dihydroxycholecalciferol ($1,25(OH)_2D_3$). Production of $1,25(OH)_2D_3$ is regulated by parathyroid hormone (PTH), phosphate, and by negative feedback. Active vitamin D is essential for the mineralization of bones and promotes the absorption of calcium ions (Ca^{2+}) and phosphate from the gut.

DEVELOPMENT OF THE KIDNEYS

The kidneys pass through three embryological developmental stages (Fig. 1.7):

1. **Pronephros:** is the most primitive system, developing in the cervical region of the embryo during the fourth week of gestation. It is nonfunctional and regresses soon after its formation, leaving behind a nephritic duct
2. **Mesonephros:** develops in the lumbar region and functions for a short period. It consists of excretory tubules with their own collecting ducts known as mesonephric ducts. These drain into the nephritic ducts
3. **Metanephros:** develops in the sacral region at approximately 5 weeks' gestation and eventually forms the final adult kidneys. It becomes functional in the latter half of the pregnancy.

The functional unit of the kidney – the nephron develops from the fusion of the:

- **Metanephric blastema,** which develops from the nephrogenic cord (part of the intermediate mesoderm). This forms the nephron tubular system from the glomerulus to the distal tubule
- **Ureteric bud,** which is an outgrowth of the mesonephric duct. This eventually dilates and splits to form the renal pelvis, calyces and collecting tubules.

The mesonephric tissue forms a cap over the ureteric bud (ampulla), which grows towards the metanephric

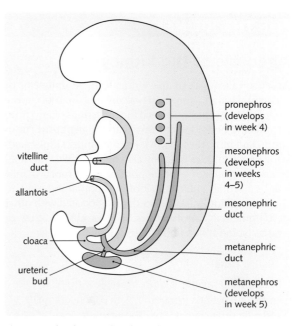

Fig. 1.7 The three embryological renal stages: pronephros, mesonephros and metanephros.

blastoma, dilates and divides repeatedly. This eventually forms the pelvis, the major and minor calyces and the collecting ducts of the kidneys. The ampulla differentiates into the nephron once fusion with the metanephric blastema is complete. A solid clump of cells near the differentiating ampulla is converted into a vesicle and fuses with the ampulla to eventually become a web of capillaries known as the glomerulus.

The metanephros initially relies on the pelvic branches of the aorta for its blood supply. Later on, the kidney ascends to the lumbar region and its primary blood supply is from the renal arteries, which branch from the aorta. Finally, the hilum of the kidney rotates from its anterior position to rest medially.

The ureters develop from the part of the ureteric bud between the pelvis and the vesicourethral canal (this develops from part of the hindgut known as the cloaca). They drain into the mesonephric ducts and the urogenital sinus. The urinary bladder develops from the mesoderm, and its epithelium is derived from both the mesoderm (the mesonephric ducts) and the endoderm (vesicourethral canal). This is summarized in Fig. 1.8.

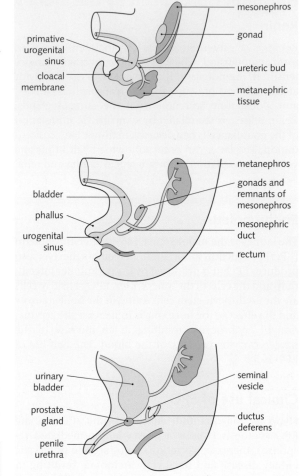

Fig. 1.8 Development of the kidneys, ureters and bladder.

HINTS AND TIPS

The kidneys and the urinary system both develop from the intermediate mesoderm at the back of the fetal abdominal cavity.

CONGENITAL ABNORMALITIES OF THE KIDNEY

Agenesis of the kidney

Absence (agenesis) of the kidney can be unilateral or bilateral. Unilateral agenesis occurs in 1 in 1000 of the population. Agenesis occurs if the collecting system (from the ureteric buds) fails to fuse with the nephrons (from the metanephric mesoderm). The remaining kidney gradually hypertrophies but may also be abnormal with malrotation, ectopia or hydronephrosis. Renal function may still be normal. There is risk of infection and trauma to the solitary kidney. This disorder is associated with other developmental abnormalities such as absent testes or ovaries, spina bifida and congenital heart disease.

Clinical Note

Bilateral renal agenesis is incompatible with life. It is also known as Potter's syndrome, with oligohydramnios and pulmonary hypoplasia. The infant has low-set ears, a flattened nose and wide-set eyes.

Hypoplasia

The kidneys develop inadequately and are consequently smaller than average. This is a rare disorder, affecting one or both kidneys, which are prone to infection and stone formation. It may also cause secondary hypertension.

Ectopic kidney

The incidence of ectopic kidney is 1 in 800. The kidney does not ascend fully into the abdomen, so remains lower than usual. If it remains in the pelvis, it is called a 'pelvic kidney'. It is usually unilateral and, the lower the kidney, the more abnormal it is. As a result of the abnormal positioning, the ureters can be obstructed by neighbouring structures, leading to obstructive uropathy, infection and stone formation. This disorder can also cause obstruction during birth.

Fig. 1.9   A horseshoe kidney.

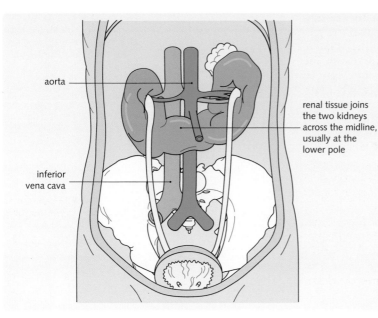

aorta

renal tissue joins
the two kidneys
across the midline,
usually at the
lower pole

inferior
vena cava

Horseshoe kidney

During their ascent during development, the kidneys may be pushed so close together that they fuse at the lower poles. The two kidneys fuse across the midline, usually at their lower poles, by renal tissue or a fibrous band (Fig. 1.9). The incidence of horseshoe kidney is between 1 in 600 and 1 in 1800, and is more common in boys than girls. The horseshoe kidney is usually lower than normal because the inferior mesenteric artery limits its ascent. It can also be malrotated and is prone to reflux, obstruction, infection and stone formation.

The glomerulus ⓶

By the end of the chapter you should be able to:
* Describe the structure of the glomerular filter
* Explain how the molecular size and charge of particles affects filtration
* Define clearance. Explain how it is measured and what its units are
* Describe how to measure the glomerular filtration rate and renal blood flow. Discuss how this varies with age
* State the four variables commonly used to estimate the glomerular filtration rate.
* Define autoregulation and explain how it is achieved
* Classify glomerular disease
* Discuss the main clinical syndromes associated with glomerular disease, giving examples of typical clinical manifestations
* Explain how acute nephritic syndrome differs from nephrotic syndrome
* State four systemic diseases associated with glomerulonephropathy

GLOMERULAR STRUCTURE AND FUNCTION

Structure of the glomerular filter

The renal corpuscle consists of a ball of capillaries, called the glomerulus, invaginated into the start of the nephron, the Bowman's capsule. This is where the first stage of urine production takes place. Plasma is filtered through the glomerular capillary wall into the Bowman's capsule. The composition of the plasma ultrafiltrate that enters the Bowman's capsule depends on the filtration barrier, which has three layers (Fig. 2.1):

1. The endothelial cells of the glomerular capillary
2. A basement membrane
3. The epithelial cells of Bowman's capsule.

Endothelial cells

The endothelial cells lining the glomerular capillaries are thin and flat with a large nucleus. The cells are perforated by numerous fenestrae (pores), which have a diameter of 60 nm. This allows plasma components to cross the vessel wall, but not blood cells or platelets.

Basement membrane

The basement membrane is a continuous layer of connective tissue and glycoproteins. It is a non-cellular structure that prevents any large molecules from being filtered.

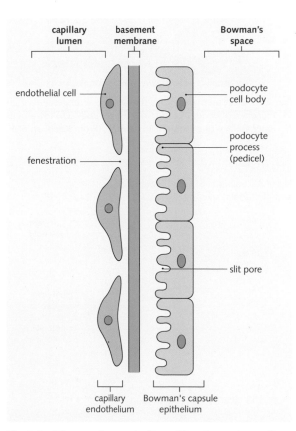

Fig. 2.1 Microscopic organization of the glomerular capillary membrane.

Epithelial lining

The epithelial lining of Bowman's capsule consists of a single layer of cells (podocytes), which rest on the basement membrane. The podocytes have large extensions or trabeculae, which extend out from the cell body and are embedded in the basement membrane surrounding a capillary. Small processes called pedicels extend out from the trabeculae and interdigitate extensively with the pedicels of adjacent trabeculae. This leads to the formation of slit pores, which control the movement of substances through the final layer of the filter. The podocytes have a well-developed Golgi apparatus, used to produce and maintain the glomerular basement membrane. Podocytes can also be involved in phagocytosis of macromolecules (Figs 2.1 and 2.2).

Mesangium

The mesangium is also part of the renal corpuscle and consists of two components:

1. Mesangial cells
2. Mesangial matrix.

The mesangial cells surround the glomerular capillaries and have a function similar to monocytes. They provide structural support for the capillaries, exhibit phagocytic activity, secrete extracellular matrix, and secrete prostaglandins. The cells are contractile, which helps regulate blood flow through the glomerular capillaries (Fig. 2.3).

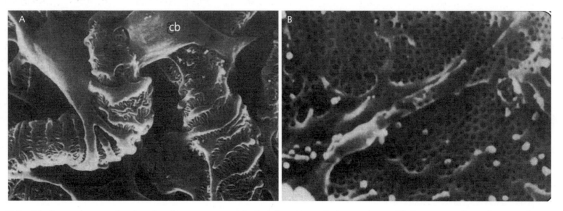

Fig. 2.2 Electron micrographs showing the arrangement of podocytes and glomerular capillaries as seen from Bowman's capsule. (A) Processes of podocytes run from the cell body (cb) towards the capillaries where they ultimately split into foot processes (pedicels). (B) Inner surface of a glomerular capillary. (From Koeppen BM, Stanton B, 1996. Renal physiology, 2nd edn. Mosby Year Book.)

Fig. 2.3 Location of extraglomerular and glomerular mesangial cells.

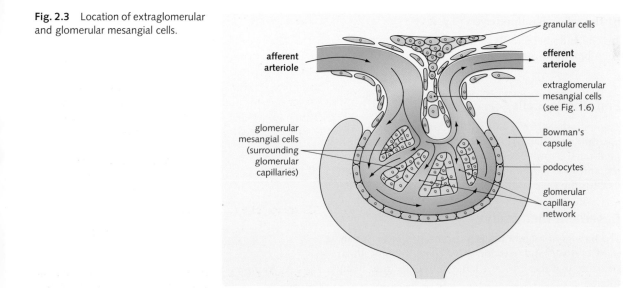

Process of glomerular filtration

This is a passive process that involves the flow of a solvent through a filter. The glomerular filter allows only low-molecular-weight substances in plasma to pass through it, forming the glomerular ultrafiltrate.

Molecular size and electrical charge

Molecular weight is the main factor in determining whether a substance is filtered or remains in the capillaries. The maximum molecular weight of substances able to pass through the filter is 70 kDa. Any molecule with a molecular weight of less than 70 kDa passes freely through the filter (e.g. glucose, amino acids, Na^+, urea, K^+). The shape and electrochemical charge of macromolecules also affect filterability. All three layers of the filter are coated with anions and these repel negatively charged macromolecules. Smaller, positively charged molecules pass through the filtration barriers relatively easily, unless they are protein-bound.

Albumin has a molecular weight of 69 kDa and is a negatively charged protein. Only very tiny amounts pass through the glomerular filter because of the repelling effect of its negative charge, and all of this is reabsorbed in the proximal tubule. A total of 30 g of protein a day enters the renal lymph vessels. Significant amounts of protein in the urine (proteinuria) are usually indicative of damage to the glomerular filter.

Glomerular filtration rate

The glomerular filtration rate (GFR) is the amount of filtrate that is produced from the blood flowing through the glomerulus per unit time.

- Normal GFR is 90–120 mL/min/1.73 m^2 (i.e. corrected for body surface area)
- The total amount filtered is 180 L/day.

The glomerular filtrate normally:

- Contains no blood cells or platelets
- Contains virtually no protein
- Is composed mostly of organic solutes with a low molecular weight and inorganic ions.

Forces governing tissue fluid formation

The movement of fluid between plasma and tissue fluid is determined by Starling's forces:

- Hydrostatic pressure (due to water)
- Colloid osmotic (oncotic) pressure (due to protein).

Changes in these forces alter the GFR. The following factors affect tissue fluid formation:

- At the arteriole end of the capillary, hydrostatic pressure is greater than colloid oncotic pressure as a result of resistance to flow due to the narrowing of the vessel, and fluid is forced out of the capillary
- As the fluid moves out of capillaries via the highly permeable wall, oncotic pressure increases and the pressure forces are reversed (most apparent at the venous end of the capillary) so there is net movement of fluid back into the capillaries.

Forces governing glomerular filtration rate

GFR is also driven by Starling's forces. However, in the renal vascular bed the surface area of the glomerular capillaries is much larger than that of normal capillary beds, so there is less resistance to flow. The hydrostatic pressure falls less along the length of the capillary because the efferent arterioles, which act as secondary resistance vessels, maintain a constant pressure along the entire length of the glomerular capillary.

Tissue fluid in a vascular bed is the equivalent of glomerular filtrate in Bowman's space, produced as a result of the glomerular capillary hydrostatic pressure (50 mmHg). This is opposed by the hydrostatic pressure in Bowman's capsule (12 mmHg) and the colloid oncotic pressure (25 mmHg) within the capillary. When these forces are equal the filtration equilibrium is reached, with very little fluid movement after this.

Fluid is reabsorbed into the peritubular capillaries as a result of high colloid oncotic pressure (35 mmHg) and low hydrostatic pressure. This reabsorption causes a fall in colloid oncotic pressure as plasma proteins become diluted.

The pressures controlling glomerular filtration into Bowman's capsule are illustrated in Fig. 2.4 and the composition of the glomerular filtrate is shown in Fig. 2.5.

Measurement of glomerular filtration rate

Clearance

Clearance (C) is the volume of plasma that is cleared of a substance in a unit time. It is a measure of the kidney's ability to remove a substance from the plasma and excrete it. The clearance of a substance x is:

$$\text{Clearance of } \chi \text{ (mL/min)} C_x = \frac{U_x \times \text{urine flow rate (mL/min)} V}{P_x}$$

where U_x = urine concentration of χ (mg/mL), V = urine flow rate (mL/min), P_x = plasma concentration of χ (mg/mL).

Clearance of a substance will provide an accurate estimate of the glomerular filtration rate (GFR) if that

Fig. 2.4 Pressures controlling glomerular filtration into Bowman's capsule. A, Hydrostatic pressure of glomerular capillary = 50 mmHg; B, hydrostatic pressure in Bowman's space = 12 mmHg (increases fluid uptake into capillary); C, oncotic pressure of glomerular capillary = 25 mmHg (increases fluid uptake into capillary).

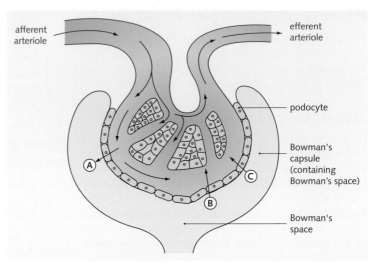

Fig. 2.5 Composition of glomerular filtrate.

Component	Glomerular filtrate
Na^+ (mmol/L)	142
K^+ (mmol/L)	4.0
Cl^- (mmol/L)	113
HCO_3^- (mmol/L)	28–30
glucose (mmol/L)	5.9
protein (g/100 mL)	0.02

$$\text{Phosphocreatine} + \text{ADP} \xrightarrow{\text{creatine phosphokinase}}$$
$$\text{creatine} + \text{ATP}$$
$$\text{Creatine} + H_2O \longrightarrow \text{creatinine}$$

Like inulin, creatinine is filtered freely and is not affected or produced by the kidney. A small contribution to the clearance of creatinine comes from tubular secretion, however with this caveat, creatinine clearance approximates to GRF. Plasma creatinine is commonly used as a marker of renal function since plasma creatinine levels will only vary with renal function as long as muscle mass and metabolism are stable. It has a reciprocal relationship with GFR (see Fig. 2.6).

substance 'follows' the filtrate without being altered by the kidney (i.e. is not reabsorbed, secreted, synthesized or metabolized by the kidney). Inulin is such a substance:

- It is a polysaccharide of molecular weight 5500
- It is not normally found within the body, so is introduced into the body by injection or intravenous infusion
- It passes into the glomerular filtrate but is not reabsorbed, secreted, synthesized or metabolized by the kidney – so all inulin filtered by the glomerulus is excreted in the urine. Inulin clearance can be used to assess glomerular function in disease.

Inulin clearance is equal to the GFR, i.e. 120 mL/min/1.73 m² body surface area (this varies with body size). GFR is widely accepted as the best measure of kidney function; however, it is difficult to measure since techniques such as inulin clearance are complicated and cannot be used to assess GFR in routine clinical practice. Instead, creatinine clearance can be used as an estimate of GFR. Creatinine is found in the body; it is produced during muscle metabolism:

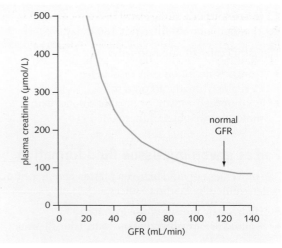

Fig. 2.6 Relation of plasma creatinine and glomerular filtration rate (GFR). Normal GFR is typically 90–120 mL/min. (From Koeppen BM, Stanton B, 1996. Renal physiology, 2nd edn. Mosby Year Book.)

Estimated glomerular filtration rate (eGFR)

The exact relationship between plasma creatinine and GFR depends upon muscle mass and therefore age, sex and size, thus plasma creatinine levels alone cannot be used as an accurate predictor of renal function. Instead the GFR may be estimated from the plasma creatinine using a formula, the most commonly used of which is the Modification of Diet in Renal Disease (MDRD) equation.

Clinical Note

MDRD eGFR is calculated from the creatinine level of the patient making an adjustment for age, sex and race.

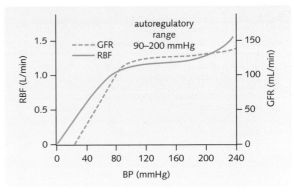

Fig. 2.8   Autoregulation of glomerular filtration rate (GFR) and renal blood flow (RBF).

Regulation of renal blood flow and glomerular filtration rate

- Renal blood flow is 1100 mL/min (renal plasma flow is 600 mL/min)
- GFR is 120 mL/min/1.73 m^2.

Both remain fairly constant because of autoregulation, which involves changes in tone of the afferent and efferent arterioles (Fig. 2.7). Over the autoregulatory range of perfusion pressures (90–200 mmHg), blood flow is independent of perfusion pressure so, as the perfusion pressure increases, resistance to flow increases (Fig. 2.8). Two mechanisms are involved in autoregulation:

1. Myogenic mechanism
2. Tubuloglomerular feedback mechanism.

Myogenic mechanism

An increase in pressure (caused by an increase in blood flow) stimulates stretch receptors in smooth muscle fibres in the vessel wall. This causes reflex contraction of smooth muscle fibres, resulting in vessel vasoconstriction. There is an increased resistance to flow so, overall, renal blood flow remains constant.

Tubuloglomerular feedback mechanism

When GFR increases, the increased flow through the tubules leads to proportionally less NaCl being reabsorbed. Hence, when the filtrate reaches the distal convoluted tubule it has a higher NaCl concentration. This is the trigger for the tubuloglomerular feedback mechanism which has three components within the juxtaglomerular apparatus:

1. The macula densa cells of the distal convoluted tubule epithelium. These detect osmolality or the rate of Na$^+$ or Cl$^-$ movement into the cells. The higher the flow of the filtrate the higher the Na$^+$ concentration in the cells
2. A signal is sent via the juxtaglomerular cells, triggered by a change in the NaCl concentration of distal tubular fluid
3. Angiotensin II or prostaglandins (see Chapter 4) act to vasoconstrict the smooth muscle of the adjacent

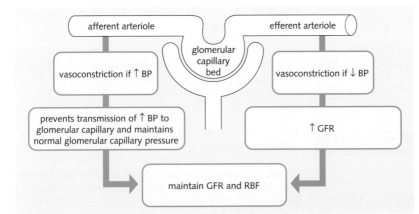

Fig. 2.7   The regulation of renal blood flow (RBF) and glomerular filtration rate (GFR) by vasoconstriction of arterioles.

Fig. 2.9 Vasoactive substances found in the blood vessel walls.

Vasodilator	Vasoconstrictor
prostaglandins (PGs)	adenosine
nitric oxide (NO)	angiotensin II
dopamine (DA)	antidiuretic hormone (ADH)
Bradykinin	endothelin
	norepinephrine (NE)

afferent arterioles and therefore decrease renal plasma flow, which in turn reduces GFR.

This mechanism maintains a constant GFR, thus preventing nephron overload because a high NaCl load decreases the filtration capacity of that nephron. A number of factors can modulate the sensitivity of the tubuloglomerular feedback mechanism including ANP and NO (decrease sensitivity) and Angiotensin II (increase sensitivity).

HINTS AND TIPS

Autoregulation of glomerular filtration relies on changes in resistance, primarily in the afferent arterioles.

Renal blood flow and systemic blood pressure

Glomerular filtration and renal blood flow remain relatively constant over a wide physiological range of blood pressure due to autoregulation. For example, in acute severe haemorrhage increased sympathetic activity leads to vasoconstriction and consequently decreased blood flow. However, in response intrarenal vasodilator prostaglandins are produced to prevent excessive vasoconstriction within the kidney and renal perfusion is thus maintained.

Regulation of GFR involves other vasoactive substances, which are found in the walls of blood vessels. These are summarized in Fig. 2.9.

DISEASES OF THE GLOMERULUS

Overview

Glomerular disease can be classified as:

- Hereditary (e.g. Alport's and Fabry's syndromes)
- Primary (most common): disease process originates from the glomerulus
- Secondary to systemic diseases: e.g. systemic lupus erythematosus (SLE), diabetes mellitus, bacterial endocarditis.

Disease of the glomerulus is frequently called a glomerulonephritis. Glomerulonephritis can result in clinical presentation with either the nephritic syndrome (haematuria with or without proteinuria salt and water retention and hypertension), or the nephrotic syndrome (heavy proteinuria sufficient to cause a low serum albumin, oedema and hypercholesterolaemia). Presentation can be acute, or chronic, rapidly or slowly progressive and may lead to chronic kidney disease. Glomerulonephritis can be asymptomatic.

Clinical Note

Four structures within the glomerulus are prone to damage:
- Capillary endothelial cell lining
- Glomerular basement membrane
- Mesangium supporting the capillaries
- Podocytes on the outer surface of the capillary
When damage occurs to the glomerulus, it results in invisible and painless haematuria and proteinuria.

The mechanisms of glomerular injury

Circulating immune complex nephritis

This is the most common mechanism of immune-mediated damage. Immune complexes form outside the kidney and become trapped in the glomerulus after travelling to the kidney via the renal circulation (Fig. 2.10B). The antigen can be:

- Exogenous: bacteria (e.g. group A streptococci), viruses (surface antigen of hepatitis B, hepatitis C virus antigen), tumour antigens
- Endogenous: e.g. DNA in SLE.

When trapped in the glomerulus, the immune complexes activate the classical complement pathway, causing acute inflammation of the glomerulus. Immunofluorescence microscopy demonstrates immunoglobulin deposits along the basement membrane and/or in the mesangium. These increase vascular permeability.

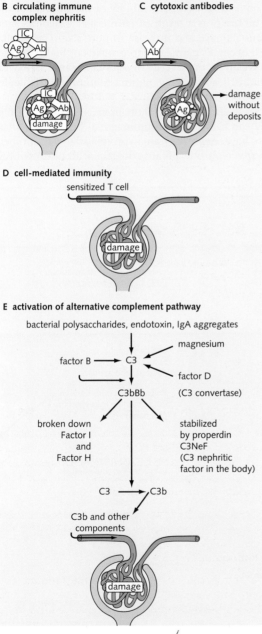

A in situ immune complex deposition

glomerulus

IC
Ag Ab — bowman's capsule
damage

B circulating immune complex nephritis

IC
Ag Ab

IC
Ag Ab
damage

C cytotoxic antibodies

Ab

Ag
damage without deposits

D cell-mediated immunity

sensitized T cell

damage

E activation of alternative complement pathway

bacterial polysaccharides, endotoxin, IgA aggregates

factor B ⟶ C3 ⟵ magnesium

⟵ factor D

C3bBb (C3 convertase)

broken down
Factor I and Factor H

stabilized by properdin C3NeF (C3 nephritic factor in the body)

C3 ⟶ C3b

C3b and other components

damage

Fig. 2.10 (A–E) The five mechanisms of immune complex renal disease. Ab, antibody; Ag, antigen; IC, immune complex.

In situ immune complex deposition

Antigen–antibody immune complexes form within the kidney when antibodies react with intrinsic or planted antigens within the glomerulus (Fig. 2.10A).

Antiglomerular basement membrane (anti-GBM) disease is an example of reaction to intrinsic antigens. Antibodies are formed against an antigen in the GBM, to form a complex which stimulates the complement cascade. This damages the glomerulus and leads to rapidly progressing renal failure. The anti-GBM antibodies also attack the basement membrane of the alveoli in the lungs. The triad of anti-GBM antibodies, GN and pulmonary haemorrhage is known as Goodpasture's syndrome.

Reaction to planted antigens occurs when circulating antigens are deposited within the glomerulus. They can be:

- Exogenous: e.g. bacteria (e.g. group A ß-haemolytic streptococci, (this may also cause circulating immune complex nephritis)), bacterial products (endostreptosin), viruses, parasites and drugs
- Endogenous: e.g. anti-DNA antibodies react with circulating DNA (as seen in SLE).

Cell-mediated immunity

Sensitized T cells from cell-mediated immune reactions play a role in the progression of acute GN to chronic GN (Fig. 2.10D). Glomerular damage is thought to be mediated by macrophages and T lymphocytes.

Activation of alternative complement pathway

Bacterial polysaccharides, endotoxins, and IgA aggregates can stimulate the alternative complement pathway – the products of which deposit in the glomeruli, impairing glomerular function (Fig. 2.10E). This occurs in membranoproliferative GN.

Cytotoxic antibodies

Antibodies to glomerular cell antigens cause damage without the formation and deposition of immune complexes (Fig. 2.10C). This is uncommon. An example would be antibody fixing to mesangial cells, resulting in complement-mediated mesangiolysis and mesangial cell proliferation.

Clinical manifestations of glomerular disease

Glomerular disease usually presents in one of the following five ways (Fig. 2.11):

1. Asymptomatic haematuria and proteinuria
2. Nephrotic syndrome
3. Acute nephritic syndrome
4. Rapidly progressive glomerular disease
5. Chronic kidney disease.

Asymptomatic haematuria

Haematuria due to glomerular disease is often invisible and painless and can be continuous or intermittent. Glomerular disease can also result in visible haematuria. Primary and secondary causes are summarized in Fig. 2.11. It should be noted that heavy exercise can result in haemoglobinuria (not haematuria).

Asymptomatic proteinuria

This is characterized by proteinuria (usually 0.3–3 g protein daily) with no other symptoms. Possible causes are summarized in Fig. 2.11.

Nephrotic syndrome

This is characterized by:

- Proteinuria (typically > 3 g/24 h) – sufficient to cause:
- Hypoalbuminaemia (serum albumin typically < 25 g/L) – sufficient to cause:
- Oedema
- Hyperlipidaemia (increased hepatic lipoprotein synthesis secondary to protein losses).

There is increased permeability of the glomerular filter to albumin as a result of glomerular basement membrane damage and increase in pore size. The capillary wall becomes permeable to proteins of higher molecular weight as the severity of injury increases. Heavy proteinuria leads to low plasma albumin and therefore tissue oedema.

In an adult, a loss of more than 3–5 g of albumin per day can cause hypoalbuminaemia, but some patients can have nephrotic-range proteinuria without being overtly nephrotic, because the rate of albumin synthesis

Fig. 2.11 Summary of types of glomerular disease and their clinical presentation.

Clinical presentation	Primary glomerular cause	Secondary cause
Asymptomatic haematuria	Mesangial IgA glomerulonephritis (GN) other GN Exercise-induced haemoglobinuria	Henoch-Schönlein purpura (HSP) systemic lupus erythematosus (SLE) bacterial endocarditis
Asymptomatic proteinuria	Mesangial capillary GN any other GN focal segmental glomerulosclerosis shunt nephritis any cause of renal scarring	HSP SLE SLE Bacterial endocarditis Polyarteritis nodosa severe long-standing hypertension pregnancy
Acute nephritic syndrome	Post-streptococcal GN non-streptococcal GN rapidly progressive GN focal proliferative GN mesangial IgA GN	SLE Microscopic polyangiitis Wegener's granulomatosis
Nephrotic syndrome	Minimal change disease Membranous glomerulonephropathy membranoproliferative GN focal segmental glomerulosclerosis	HSP SLE Tumour amyloid Diabetes mellitus drugs (e.g. penicillamine, gold) Bacterial endocarditis congenital nephrotic syndrome
Chronic kidney disease glomerulosclerosis	This develops as a long-term consequence of any of above diseases	

compensates for the albumin loss. A limited amount of filtered protein can be reabsorbed by endocytosis, but if this is exceeded, protein is lost in the urine. A normal albumin concentration within the capillary maintains the colloid osmotic pressure and when this is decreased, less fluid moves back into the capillaries, causing oedema in the peripheral tissues. The decreased circulating volume stimulates the renin–angiotensin–aldosterone system, leading to further sodium and water retention, and further oedema.

Other proteins can be lost from the plasma, including immunoglobulins and proteins controlling coagulation. Complications of nephrotic syndrome include:

- Immunosuppression: increases risk of infection
- Hypercoagulable state: increases risk of deep vein thrombosis, pulmonary embolus and renal vein thrombosis
- Hyperlipidaemia: increases risk of vascular disease and ischaemic heart disease.

Management includes:

- Blood pressure control
- Reduction of proteinuria, using angiotensin-converting enzyme (ACE) inhibitors
- Control of hyperlipidaemia
- Anticoagulation if hypercoagulable (risk of thrombosis increases as albumin decreases)
- Treatment of underlying causes when possible, e.g. in minimal change disease high-dose corticosteroid therapy will eliminate proteinuria in up to 90% of cases.

Primary and secondary causes are summarized in Fig. 2.11.

Acute nephritic syndrome

The symptoms and signs include:

- Oliguria/anuria
- Hypertension
- Fluid retention – seen as facial oedema
- Haematuria – microscopic or macroscopic
- Uraemia
- Proteinuria.

Patients might also complain of loin pain, headache and general malaise. Primary and secondary causes of acute nephritic syndrome are summarized in Fig. 2.11.

HINTS AND TIPS

Remember the difference between nephrotic and nephritic syndromes. **Nephrotic** syndrome is characterized by the massive loss of protein causing

the various complications. In acute **nephritic** syndrome there may be some proteinuria but more importantly there is haematuria, oliguria and hypertension.

Rapidly progressive GN

Rapidly progressive GN, or crescentic GN, occurs when there is severe glomerular injury. It presents with haematuria, oliguria and hypertension, eventually causing renal failure. This may be seen in a renal vasculitis such as Wegner's granulomatosis or microscopic polyangiitis.

Chronic kidney disease (CKD)

Chronic glomerulonephritis causes CKD as a result of progressive nephron loss. The kidney shrinks, with cortical thinning and granular scarring. Histological examination of chronic glomerulonephritis reveals:

- Glomeruli hyalinization
- Tubular atrophy
- Interstitial fibrosis.

This is often asymptomatic in the early stages. Later, symptoms of CKD develop as waste products accumulate and erythropoietin or vitamin D production is reduced. Symptoms and signs of CKD (discussed in detail in Chapter 7) include:

- Hypertension
- Salt and water retention causing oedema
- Anaemia
- Nausea, vomiting, diarrhoea
- Gastrointestinal bleeding
- Itching
- Polyuria and nocturia
- Lethargy
- Paraesthesiae (due to polyneuropathy)
- Mental slowing and clouding of consciousness (terminal stage).

In extreme cases, oliguria results. Dialysis or renal transplantation are effective treatments. The glomerular causes of CKD are given in Fig. 2.11, however, when advanced it is usually not possible to determine the nature of the initial insult.

HINTS AND TIPS

Scarring of the glomerulus is known as glomerulosclerosis, the histological hallmark of CKD.

Primary glomerulonephritis typically presenting with heavy proteinuria or the nephrotic syndrome

Minimal change disease

This is the most common cause of nephrotic syndrome in children under the age of 6 years, and more commonly affects males. No significant renal changes are seen under the light microscope (hence the name). Electron microscopy shows podocyte fusion, i.e. foot process effacement. The cause is unknown, but potential mechanisms include a post-allergic reaction, circulating immune complexes, or altered T-cell immunity. Treatment involves corticosteroid therapy and ciclosporin or cyclophosphamide (if resistant). The prognosis is good in children and variable in adults, but usually good with it only very rarely causing end-stage renal failure.

Membranous glomerulonephropathy

This is a chronic disease characterized by:

- Subepithelial deposition of immune complexes
- Basement membrane thickening.

It accounts for 40% of adult nephrotic syndrome and is more common in males. Causes are idiopathic (85%), primary or secondary. Secondary causes include:

- Infections: syphilis, malaria, hepatitis B
- Tumours: melanoma, carcinoma of the bronchus, lymphoma
- Drugs: penicillamine, heroin, mercury, gold
- Systemic illnesses: SLE.

Histological examination reveals widespread glomerular basement thickening caused by immunoglobulin deposition. Over time, the abnormal excess mesangial matrix causes hyalinization of the glomerulus and death of individual nephrons. Treatment could involve immunosuppressants. Prognosis depends on the cause; 30% of idiopathic cases develop CKD and require dialysis or transplantation. In secondary membranous glomerulonephropathy, treatment of underlying disease causes disease remission.

Clinical Note

- Membranous GN is the most common cause of nephrotic syndrome in older patients
- Minimal change GN is the most common cause of nephrotic syndrome in children.

Focal segmental glomerulosclerosis

This accounts for 10% of childhood and up to 30% of cases of adult nephrotic syndrome. It is more common in males and its causes are:

- Altered cellular immunity
- Intravenous heroin use
- Acquired immune deficiency syndrome
- Reaction to chronic proteinuria
- Idiopathic.

Histological examination reveals focal collapse and sclerosis, with hyaline deposits in glomerular segments. Presentation is with proteinuria or nephrotic syndrome, later developing haematuria and hypertension. Most develop CKD within 10 years. Treatment of the idiopathic form might involve steroids, cyclophosphamide, ciclosporin, dialysis and renal transplantation. Recurrence can be seen after a renal transplant.

Primary glomerulonephritis typically presenting with the nephritic syndrome

IgA nephropathy (Berger's disease)

This is the most common primary glomerular disease worldwide, causing recurrent haematuria. There is some association with geographical location (more common in France, Australia and Singapore) and human leucocyte antigen (HLA) DR4. It typically affects young men after an upper respiratory tract infection. Presentation is with microscopic haematuria and proteinuria and renal impairment. There is hypertension and plasma IgA levels are raised. Histologically IgA and C3 deposits are seen in the mesangium of all the glomeruli, with some mesangial proliferation (this is similar to the histological picture seen in HSP). Eventually, there is sclerosis of the damaged segment. There is no effective treatment. Patients with late onset, proteinuria, increased blood pressure and increased creatinine at presentation have a worse prognosis – up to 20% of patients develop advanced CKD.

Rapidly progressive (crescentic) glomerulonephritis

This results in severe glomerular injury. Histologically, glomerular injury results in leakage of fibrin, which stimulates epithelial cells and macrophages within Bowman's capsule to proliferate and form crescent-shaped masses, reducing glomerular blood supply. It can be seen as part of systemic illnesses such as SLE, Wegener's granulomatosis and microscopic polyangiitis. As the name suggests, the disease progresses rapidly and there is a loss of renal function within days to weeks. Prompt diagnosis and treatment is therefore required to prevent hypertension, kidney scarring and renal failure. Treatment consists of high-dose steroids, immunosuppressants and plasma exchange.

Focal proliferative glomerulonephritis

Focal proliferative GN results in inflammation of some parts of some glomeruli. Its presentation is less acute. It might affect only the kidney (IgA nephropathy, see below) or be secondary to systemic illnesses such as Henoch–Schönlein purpura (HSP), Goodpasture's syndrome, subacute bacterial endocarditis, vasculitis and other connective tissue diseases (e.g. SLE). Treatment with immunosuppression can be effective. The prognosis is variable. Necrotizing GN is also often seen in malignant hypertension.

Membranoproliferative glomerulonephropathy

Also known as mesangiocapillary glomerulonephritis, this is rare. It occurs most often in children and females. It is characterized histologically by diffuse global basement membrane thickening and mesangial proliferation. It is usually primary, but can be secondary to disorders such as SLE and malaria. Primary membranoproliferative GN is classified as:

- Type I (more common): immune complexes deposit in the subendothelium, causing inflammation and capillary thickening
- Type II: caused by activation of the alternative complement pathway following an infection. Histological examination reveals thickened capillaries caused by C3 deposition.

It can present with asymptomatic haematuria or combined nephrotic/nephritic syndrome.

Secondary glomerulonephritis

Systemic disorders can cause glomerular disease. They can be:

- Immune complex mediated (e.g. SLE, HSP, bacterial endocarditis)
- Vascular (e.g. microscopic polyangiitis, Wegener's granulomatosis)
- Metabolic (e.g. diabetes mellitus, amyloidosis)
- Drug treatment (e.g. penicillamine, gold, captopril, phenytoin)
- Infections (e.g. hepatitis B, leprosy, syphilis, malaria).

Post-streptococcal glomerulonephritis

This presents 1–3 weeks following a group A ß-haemolytic streptococcal infection of the tonsils, pharynx or skin. Clinical features include proteinuria, haematuria and a low glomerular filtration rate (GFR) (this causes fluid retention, oligaemia and hypertension). All the glomeruli are involved thus resulting in a diffuse proliferative GN – 'proliferative' because there is an increase in the cellularity in the glomerulus (Fig. 2.12). Treatment is usually conservative, with antibiotics to treat any remaining infection. The prognosis is excellent in children but only 60% of adults recover completely; the rest develop hypertension or renal impairment.

Non-streptococcal glomerulonephritis

Non-streptococcal GN follows a similar process to that for post-streptococcal GN except that the causative organism is not a *Streptococcus*. It can be triggered by:

- Other bacteria (i.e. staphylococci and pneumococci)
- Parasites (*Toxoplasma gondii, Plasmodium*)
- Viruses.

Systemic lupus erythematosus

SLE is an autoimmune vasculitis characterized by antinuclear antibodies and widespread immune-complex-mediated inflammation. It is more common

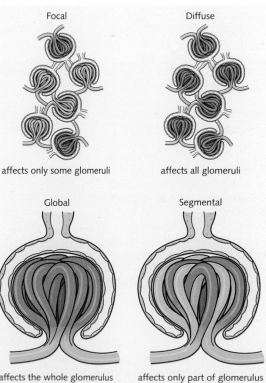

Fig. 2.12   Terminology in glomerulonephritis.

in females, Asians and if an individual is HLA B8-, DR2- or DR3-positive. It is a relapsing and remitting condition, usually diagnosed between 30 and 40 years of age. It affects many systems and organs in the body; for example, the joints, skin, heart, lungs and the kidneys (75% of cases). The renal lesions are the most important clinically and affect prognosis. Glomerular changes vary from minimal involvement to diffuse proliferative disease with:

- Immune complex deposition in glomerulus (frequently all classes of immunoglobulin and complement)
- Basement membrane thickening
- Endothelial proliferation.

This results in focal or diffuse proliferative GN, or membranous glomerulopathy. Patients present with proteinuria, oedema and hypertension. There may be extrarenal systemic symptoms. Patients may develop CKD, but the prognosis is improved with immuno-suppressive treatment (steroids, azathioprine or cyclophosphamide).

Henoch–Schönlein purpura

HSP is seen predominantly in children, affecting males more than females. It is an immune-mediated systemic vasculitis that affects many parts of the body including:

- Skin: a purpuric rash is seen over on the extensor surface of the legs, arms and buttocks
- Joints: resulting in pain
- Intestine: resulting in abdominal pain, vomiting, bleeding

- Kidney: resulting in GN (a third of patients develop glomerular lesions histologically identical to IgA nephropathy).

HSP can follow an upper respiratory tract infection. It has an excellent prognosis in children.

Bacterial endocarditis

Glomerular disease in bacterial endocarditis is caused by:

- Immune complex deposits in the glomerulus
- Embolism-mediated infarction – emboli break away from the heart valves.

The main histological diagnoses are focal, segmental and diffuse proliferative GN. Presentation is with microscopic haematuria, fluid retention and renal impairment. Renal lesions resolve on antibiotic therapy.

Diabetic glomerulosclerosis

Diabetes mellitus affects several organs including the kidneys, which are the most commonly and severely damaged organs in diabetes. Diabetic nephropathy is the most common cause of CKD requiring dialysis treatment in developed countries. Renal manifestations include nodular glomerulosclerosis and arteriosclerosis, including benign nephrosclerosis with hypertension (Fig. 2.13 presents a summary of the natural history of diabetes). Histological features can include:

- Thickening of the capillary basement membrane
- Increase in the matrix of the mesangium
- A diffuse or nodular pattern of glomerulosclerosis (also known as Kimmelstiel–Wilson syndrome)

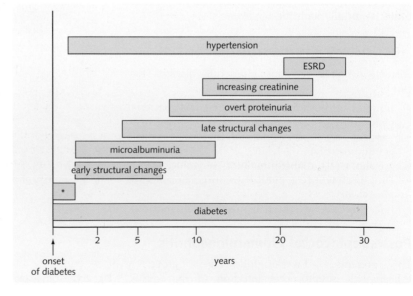

Fig. 2.13 Summary of the natural history of diabetes. 'Asterisk' (*) indicates functional changes in kidney size (increased) and short-term glomerular filtration rate (increased). ESRD, end-stage renal disease (or CKD stage 5).

- Arterial hyalinosis of both the afferent and efferent arterioles – this predisposes to vessel occlusion.

The arteries can also be affected (especially in type II diabetes) and severe atheroma in the renal artery leads to renal ischaemia and hypertension. Papillary necrosis is a recognized complication, especially in the presence of infection.

Diabetic nephropathy presents with microalbuminuria, which increases progressively to nephrotic range proteinuria (i.e. >3 g/24 h). Consequently, GFR gradually declines, leading to CKD, which can be seen in 30% of cases of insulin-dependent type 1 diabetes mellitus. It is also associated with diabetic complications elsewhere (e.g. retinopathy in the eyes). Chronic renal damage as a result of diabetes is associated and accelerated by hypertension.

Treatment includes ACE inhibitors to reduce proteinuria (these are discussed later), strict blood pressure and glycaemic control, and dialysis for stage 5 CKD.

Amyloidosis

This disorder involves deposition of amyloid (an extracellular fibrillar protein) in the glomeruli, usually within the mesangium and subendothelium, and sometimes in the subepithelial space. Deposits can also be found in the walls of the blood vessels and in the interstitium. Clinically, this results in heavy proteinuria or the nephrotic syndrome, eventually leading to CKD (due to ischaemia and glomerulosclerosis). Dialysis or transplant is required to prevent death from uraemia.

Goodpasture's syndrome

In Goodpasture's syndrome, autoantibodies to type IV collagen in the glomerular basement membrane develop, causing inflammation. Presentation is with a rapidly progressive crescentic GN and acute renal failure (ARF) and lung haemorrhage. Prognosis is poor without treatment, which involves:

- Plasma exchange (to remove the antibodies)
- Corticosteroids (to reduce inflammation).

Microscopic polyarteritis nodosa (also known as microscopic polyangiitis)

This is a necrotizing vasculitis affecting the small arteries of the body; it is more common in males. Initially, there is a focal, segmental or necrotizing GN followed by rapidly progressive GN. Histological examination reveals extensive necrosis, fibrin deposition and epithelial crescents. Microscopic polyarteritis nodosa (PAN) is associated with circulating antineutrophil cytoplasmic antibodies (ANCA), which complex with a perinuclear antigen (myeloperoxidase) in fixed neutrophils (pANCA).

Wegener's granulomatosis

This is a rare necrotizing vasculitis affecting the nose, upper respiratory tract and kidneys. It typically presents between 40 and 50 years of age. The glomerular disease is similar to that in microscopic PAN, with granuloma formation. Presentation is with asymptomatic haematuria or nephritic syndrome (focal segmental GN) or rapidly progressive GN. It is associated with ANCA, which characteristically recognizes a cytoplasmic antigen (proteinase 3) in fixed neutrophils (cANCA).

Hereditary nephritis

Alport's syndrome

This is usually X-linked, affecting mainly males (females are usually asymptomatic carriers). Autosomal dominant and autosomal recessive patterns of inheritance have also been described. An abnormality of basement membrane collagen IV is found in all patients, and they lack the Goodpasture's antigen.

Presentation is with glomerulonephritis and haematuria, ocular abnormalities and sensorineural deafness. Ocular lesions include lens dislocation, cataract and conical cornea. It is also associated with platelet dysfunction and hyperproteinaemia.

A few patients develop end-stage renal failure in childhood and adolescence. Females might have microscopic haematuria, but rarely develop end-stage renal failure. Treatment involves dialysis and/or transplantation.

Fabry's syndrome

This is a rare X-linked disorder, with a glycolipid metabolism defect due to the deficiency of galacto-sidase A. As a result, ceramide trihexoside (a glyco-sphingolipid) accumulates and is deposited in the kidneys, skin and vascular system. This disorder is associated with cardiac problems such as angina and cardiac failure – consequently, most patients die in the fifth decade of life.

The tubules and the interstitium

3

Objectives

By the end of the chapter you should be able to:
- Define reabsorption, secretion and excretion
- Outline the difference between primary and secondary active transport
- State the normal pH range. Outline how and why it is tightly controlled
- Explain what a 'buffer' is, and name the main buffering system in the body and describe how it works
- Explain how metabolic acidosis and metabolic alkalosis are differentiated by arterial blood gas results and give an outline of how you would correct each of them
- Explain the relation between plasma calcium and phosphate
- Describe the influence of three factors involved in their regulation
- List five drugs used in the management of hyperkalaemia and state how they work
- Understand the countercurrent mechanism of the loop of Henle
- Briefly describe the synthesis, storage and function of antidiuretic hormone (ADH)
- Describe how the kidneys' ability to concentrate or dilute urine is altered in disease
- List the causes and the clinical presentation of syndrome of inappropriate ADH secretion (SIADH)
- Distinguish the two types of diabetes insipidus and explain how they differ
- State how the tubules are damaged in ATN and describe rhabdomyolysis
- List the predisposing factors for pyelonephritis
- Give three mechanisms by which multiple myeloma causes damage to the kidney

OVERVIEW

This chapter considers the convoluted tubules, loop of Henle, collecting duct and the interstitium between these tubules. The ultrafiltrate produced from the glomerular filter has a similar composition to plasma. The tubules and the interstitium are considered to act together, modifying the ultrafiltrate through reabsorption and secretion to produce the final urine. This process is important in maintaining a normal homeostasis of many ions in the body.

TRANSPORT PROCESSES IN THE RENAL TUBULE

Reabsorption, secretion and excretion are defined as follows:

- **Reabsorption**: the movement of a substance from the tubular fluid back into the circulation
- **Secretion**: the movement of substances from the blood into the tubular fluid via tubular cells (active transport) or intercellular spaces (passive process)
- **Excretion**: the removal of waste products from the blood and the net result of filtration, secretion and reabsorption of a substance.

Fig. 3.1 illustrates the processes that occur in the nephron and result in excretion of a substance. Two types of solute transport are involved:

1. Paracellular movement (between cells) across the tight junctions that connect the cells. This is driven by concentration and the electrical and osmotic gradients
2. Transcellular movement (through cells) via both the apical and basal membranes and the cell cytoplasm. Here, water follows the movement of solutes by osmosis.

Transport mechanisms

Diffusion

Diffusion is the movement of substances down their electrochemical gradient. It is a 'passive' process, as it does not require any metabolic energy or carrier molecules.

Facilitated diffusion

Like diffusion, this is also passive movement of substances along their electrochemical gradient, but it relies on a carrier molecule to transport substances across the membrane. Consequently, it is much faster than diffusion.

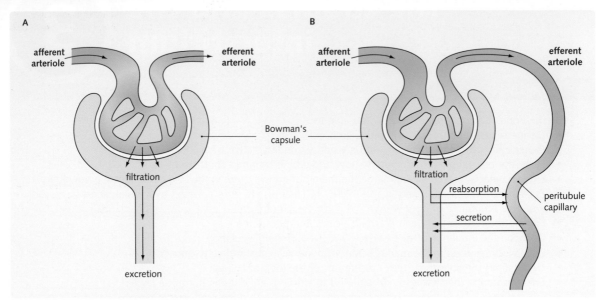

Fig. 3.1 (A, B) Processes that result in the excretion of a substance in the nephron.

Primary active transport

This is an energy-dependent process in which substances cross cell membranes against their concentration and electrochemical gradients. It involves the hydrolysis of adenosine triphosphate (ATP), which provides chemical energy for the transport mechanism.

The most important active transporter is the Na^+/K^+ ATPase pump, which is found on the basal and basolateral membranes of tubular cells. It is involved in the active transport of Na^+ from intracellular to extracellular spaces, allowing the nephron to reabsorb over 99% of the filtered Na^+. This maintains a low Na^+ concentration and a high K^+ concentration in the cell (Fig. 3.2). The other primary active transporters on the tubular cell membrane are:

- Ca^{2+} ATPase
- H^+/K^+ ATPase
- H^+ ATPase.

The ATP molecule is part of the protein structure in the primary active transporters. Energy is derived from the hydrolysis of the terminal phosphate bond of the ATP molecule to form adenosine diphosphate (ADP) and phosphate (P_i) (Fig. 3.3).

Secondary active transport

This process uses the energy produced from another process for transporting molecules (i.e. the transport of the solutes is coupled). The most important example of this mechanism involves the Na^+/K^+ ATPase pump as the driving force for the secretion and reabsorption of other solutes in which the energy is provided by the Na^+ gradient.

The Na^+/K^+ ATPase pump creates an ionic gradient across the cell membrane, which allows the energy produced from the diffusion of Na^+ into the cell as it moves along its electrochemical gradient to be used for active transport (i.e. against their electrochemical gradients) of other solutes.

Substances can move in two directions by the following processes:

- **Symport**: energy produced by the movement of Na^+ is used to transport other substances in the same direction across the cell membrane, i.e. with the Na^+ gradient (e.g. the $Na^+/K^+/Cl^-$ co-transporter in the thick ascending limb and the Na^+/glucose in the cells of the proximal tubule cells)
- **Antiport**: movement of substances against their electrochemical gradient in the opposite direction to the Na^+ gradient (e.g. the Ca^{2+}/Na^+ and the H^+/Na^+ exchangers).

These processes are carried out by specific carrier proteins embedded in the cell membrane called transporters.

- H^+/K^+ ATPase
- Proton pump
- Ca^{2+} ATPase
- Na^+/K^+ ATPase (sodium pump).

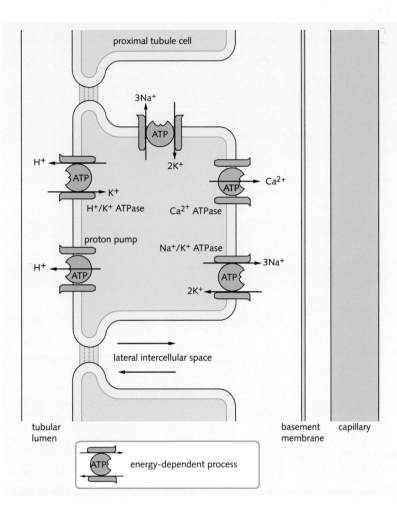

Fig. 3.2 Mechanisms of active transport in the proximal tubule cells.

proximal tubule cell

3Na⁺

ATP

2K⁺

H⁺

ATP

K⁺

H⁺/K⁺ ATPase

Ca²⁺ ATPase

Ca²⁺

proton pump

Na⁺/K⁺ ATPase

H⁺

ATP

3Na⁺

2K⁺

lateral intercellular space

tubular lumen

basement membrane

capillary

ATP   energy-dependent process

Ion channels

These are protein pores found on the epithelial cell membranes. They allow rapid transport of ions into the cell. Channels that are specific for Na^+, K^+ and Cl^- are found on the apical membrane of all the cells lining the nephron. Although transport through these channels is very fast (10^6–10^8 ions/s) there are only about 100 channels per cell, compared with the slower (100 ions/s) but more numerous active transporters (10^7 transporters per cell).

REGULATION OF BODY FLUID pH

Body fluid pH is tightly controlled because most enzyme reactions are sensitive to pH changes.

* Normal pH range is 7.35–7.45
* Normal H^+ concentration is 35–45 nmol/L.

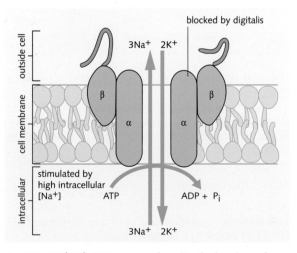

blocked by digitalis

3Na⁺   2K⁺

outside cell

cell membrane

β   β

α   α

intracellular

stimulated by high intracellular [Na⁺]   ATP   ADP + Pᵢ

3Na⁺   2K⁺

Fig. 3.3 Na^+/K^+ ATPase pump found in the basal membrane of the cells. It drives secondary active transport by maintaining a low Na^+ concentration in the cells.

Buffers

Definition

A buffer is a mixture of a weak acid (HA) and a conjugate base. It undergoes minimal pH change when either an acid or a base is added to it:

$$HA \rightleftharpoons H^+ (acid) + A^- (conjugate\ base)$$

It can also be a mixture of a weak base (BH) and conjugate acid:

$$BA \rightleftharpoons H^+ (conjugate\ acid) + B^- (base)$$

For example, if there is an increase in H^+, the equations above shift to the left so that the extra H^+ combines with the buffer and the H^+ concentration in the body falls.

Henderson-Hasselbalch equation

This equation is used to determine the pH of body fluids from the buffer concentrations. The equations below show how it is derived mathematically. K_a is the acid dissociation constant, the equilibrium constant in terms of conjugate acids and bases, proton donators, and acceptors.

$$HA \rightleftharpoons H^+ + A^-$$

Equation 1. At equilibrium:

$$K_a = \frac{[H^+][A^-]}{[HA]}$$

$$\therefore [H^+] = \frac{K_a[HA]}{[A^-]}$$

$$= \frac{K_a[acid]}{[base]}$$

Equation 2:

$$pH = -\log [H^+]$$
$$= \frac{\log 1}{[H^+]}$$
$$pK_a = -\log K_a$$
$$= \frac{\log 1}{K_a}$$

Equation 3. Combining equations 1 and 2 (the Henderson–Hasselbalch equation).

$$pH = pK_a + \log \frac{[base]}{[acid]}$$

Physiological buffers

There are several buffer systems in the different body compartments (Fig. 3.4), of which the most important is the bicarbonate buffer system.

Fig. 3.4 Buffer systems in different body compartments.

Buffer systems	Blood	ECF and CSF	ICF
HCO_3^-/CO_2	✓	✓	✓
Haemoglobin	✓		
Plasma proteins	✓		
Phosphate	✓	✓	✓
Organic phosphate			✓
Proteins		✓	✓

CSF, cerebrospinal fluid; ECF, extracellular fluid; ICF, intracellular fluid.

Bicarbonate buffer system

The bicarbonate buffer system is important in all body fluids. CO_2 and H_2O combine to form carbonic acid (H_2CO_3) in the presence of the enzyme carbonic anhydrase (CA). The H_2CO_3 then dissociates spontaneously to form bicarbonate ions (HCO_3^-) and H^+:

$$CO_2 + H_2O \underset{}{\overset{carbonic\ anhydrase}{\rightleftharpoons}} H_2CO_3 \rightleftharpoons H^+ + HCO_3^-$$

CO_2 concentration is regulated by the lungs and HCO_3^- concentration is regulated by the kidneys. Therefore, pH regulation depends equally on both these organs. Substituting this equation in the Henderson–Hasselbalch equation, we get:

$$pH = pK_a + \log \frac{[HCO_3^-]}{[H_2CO_3]}$$

The acid dissociation constant, pK_a, of the HCO_3^-/pCO_2 system = 6.1.

$[H_2CO_3]$ is determined by dissolved CO_2: $[H_2CO_3] = 0.23 \times pCO_2$ (0.23 is the CO_2 solubility coefficient at 37 °C; pCO_2 is the pressure of CO_2 in the lungs in kPa)

$$Therefore,\ pH = 6.1 + \log \frac{[HCO_3^-]}{0.23 \times pCO_2}$$

This is the key equation that can be used to relate pH, $[HCO_3^-]$ and pCO_2. Normal values are:

- $[HCO_3^-]$: 22–26 mmol/L
- pCO_2: 4.7–6.0 kPa
- pH: 7.35–7.45.

$$CO_2 + H_2O \rightleftharpoons H_2CO_3 \rightleftharpoons H^+ + HCO_3^-$$

From this you can see that if $[HCO_3^-]$ rises, $[H^+]$ will become lower, hence pH will rise. If pCO_2 rises, the pH will become lower. This relationship is calculated precisely by the Henderson-Hasselbalch equation.

Renal regulation of plasma HCO_3^-

The kidneys control the concentration of HCO_3^- in the plasma. They can only reabsorb up to a certain amount of HCO_3^- per second (T_m). If plasma HCO_3^- increases, T_m is exceeded and the kidneys cannot reabsorb all of it, some HCO_3^- is excreted until the plasma level returns to normal.

HCO_3^- reabsorption by the proximal tubule

On the apical membrane Na^+ reabsorption down its concentration gradient drives H^+ secretion into the lumen. H^+ combines with HCO_3^- ions to form H_2CO_3 (carbonic acid). Carbonic anhydrase (CA) on the brush border of the cells catalyses the dissociation of H_2CO_3 to $H_2O + CO_2$ within the tubular lumen. Both H_2O and CO_2 diffuse freely into the cell, where they re-form H_2CO_3, this process being catalysed by intracellular CA. HCO_3^- and Na^+ are actively transported out of the cell across the basolateral membrane. H^+ is secreted out of the cell into the tubular lumen and recycled to allow continuation of this cycle (Fig. 3.5). CA inhibitors suppress H^+ secretion, leading to a fall in Na^+ and HCO_3^- absorption, and thus act as a weak diuretic.

HCO_3^- reabsorption by the distal tubule

Only a small amount of HCO_3^- can be reabsorbed by the intercalated cells of the distal tubule. The Na^+

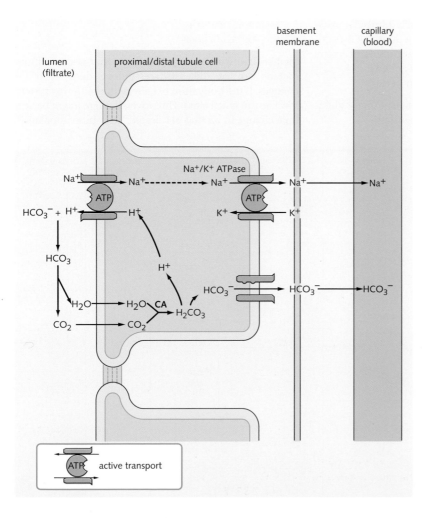

Fig. 3.5 HCO_3^- reabsorption in the proximal tubule cells. Secreted H^+ combines with HCO_3^- to form carbonic acid. This is broken down by carbonic anhydrase (CA) in the brush border to CO_2 and H_2O, which diffuse freely into the cell. The process is reversed inside the cell to re-form HCO_3^-.

gradient is insufficient so H^+ is pumped into the lumen using H^+-ATPase. Little CO_2 is produced in the lumen to enter the cell so CO_2 from the cell's own metabolism is used to create HCO_3^-, which is moved into the plasma.

Conversion of alkaline phosphate to acid phosphate – luminal buffer

Alkaline phosphate Na_2HPO_4 and acid phosphate NaH_2PO_4 are present in the plasma in the ratio of 4:1. Both are filtered at the glomerulus. Alkaline phosphate is converted to acid phosphate, mainly in the distal tubule but also in the proximal tubule. This generates Na^+ and binds H^+ in the lumen. This feeds the system already described, generating HCO_3^- for the plasma (Fig. 3.5). The buffer is more effective at a lower pH.

Ammonia secretion – luminal buffer

Deamination of glutamine in the proximal tubule yields ammonium ions (NH_4^+) and HCO_3^-. This NH_4^+ is secreted into the lumen and the HCO_3^- enters the plasma (Fig. 3.6). Fifty percent of NH_4^+ secreted into the proximal tubule is actually reabsorbed by the thick ascending limb of the loop of Henle and accumulates in the cells of the medullary interstitium (Fig. 3.7).

Acidosis increases NH_4^+ excretion because:

- Acidosis stimulates enzymes that deaminate glutamine, thereby increasing NH_4^+ synthesis

- Increased H^+ secretion results in NH_3 production, which in turn results in increased NH_4^+ in the collecting tubules. The conversion of NH_3 to NH_4^+ maintains a gradient for NH_3 secretion. In this way, excess NH_3/NH_4^+ is removed from the medulla.

Acid–base disturbances

If the pH of the blood is too high, this is called alkalaemia, which is dangerous principally because it reduces the solubility of calcium salts. The resulting hypocalcaemia causes excitation of nerves leading to tetany.

If the pH of the blood is too low, this is called acidaemia, which can lead to potassium ions being pumped out of cells in exchange for hydrogen ions through exchange channels. The resulting hyperkalaemia can cause cardiac arrhythmias.

The processes that tend to cause alkalaemia or acidaemia are respectively called alkalosis and acidosis. There are four main types:

1. Respiratory acidosis
2. Respiratory alkalosis
3. Metabolic acidosis
4. Metabolic alkalosis.

Metabolic disturbances result from changes in cellular metabolism or diet, so are independent of pCO_2 changes. If the body fluid pH alters, the buffering system mechanism is activated. Thus, overall, there might be very little change in arterial pH despite acid–base imbalance.

Fig. 3.6 Renal secretion and handling of NH_3.

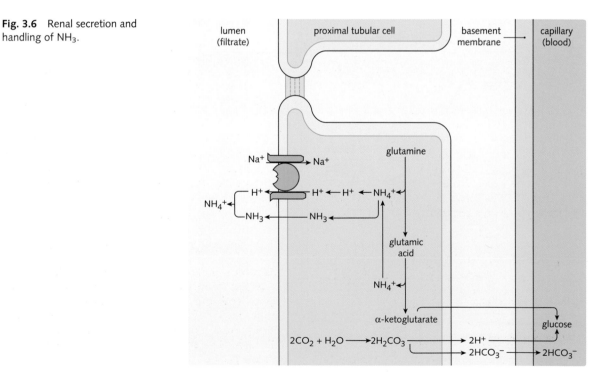

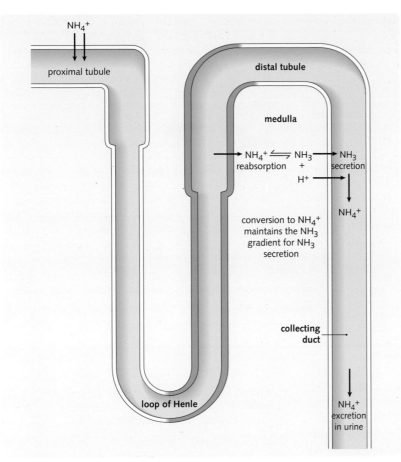

Fig. 3.7 Handling of NH_3 and NH_4^+ by nephrons.

- Compensation is the restoration of normal pH even when acid–base imbalance is still present
- Correction is the restoration of both the pH and acid–base imbalance to normal.

Arterial blood gases (ABGs) measure the pH, pO_2 and pCO_2 in an arterial blood sample. This can be used to diagnose an acid–base imbalance. The Davenport diagram is a graph of the plasma HCO_3^- versus plasma pH, used to classify acid–base disturbances (Fig. 3.8). For example, if pH = 7.2 and pCO_2 is 9.3 kPa, by looking at Fig. 3.8 it can be seen that $[HCO_3^-]$ will be raised. This corresponds to a respiratory acidosis.

Examples of acid–base disturbances

Respiratory acidosis

The causes of respiratory acidosis are:

- Chronic obstructive pulmonary disease (COPD)
- Obstruction of the airway (e.g. tumour, foreign body)

- Mechanical chest injuries
- Severe asthma
- Drugs: general anaesthetic, morphine, barbiturates (respiratory centre depressant)
- Injuries and infections to the respiratory centre in the brainstem.

ABG results show $pCO_2 > 6.0$ kPa and decreased pH. Clinically, the respiratory system cannot remove enough CO_2, so CO_2 increases together with pCO_2. Therefore the following equation is shifted to the right:

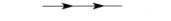

$$CO_2 + H_2O \rightleftharpoons H_2CO_3 \rightleftharpoons H^+ + HCO_3^-$$

This results in elevated $[H^+]$ and $[HCO_3^-]$. The extra H^+ results in increased H^+ secretion and increased HCO_3^- reabsorption. This restores pH, acting as a compensatory response. The acid–base disturbance is not corrected because the pCO_2 and $[HCO_3^-]$ are still high. Correction requires hyperventilation to decrease pCO_2.

Fig. 3.8 Acid and base disturbances with compensatory changes demonstrated on the Davenport diagram.

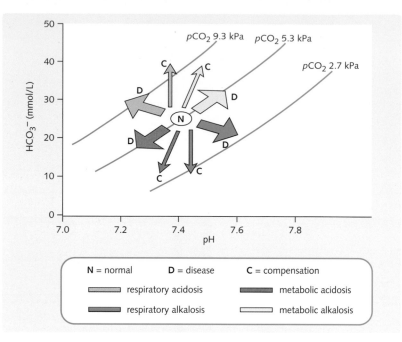

N = normal   D = disease   C = compensation

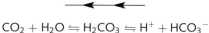 respiratory acidosis   metabolic acidosis

respiratory alkalosis   metabolic alkalosis

Respiratory alkalosis

The causes of respiratory alkalosis are:

- Decreased pO_2, which is detected by chemoreceptors in the carotid body resulting in hyperventilation and decreased pCO_2
- High altitude
- Fever
- Brainstem damage resulting in hyperventilation
- Hysterical overbreathing.

The ABG results show a $pCO_2 < 4.7$ kPa and an elevated pH. Clinically too much CO_2 is removed by the respiratory system. Therefore the following equation is shifted to the left:

$$CO_2 + H_2O \leftharpoons H_2CO_3 \leftharpoons H^+ + HCO_3^-$$

This causes [H^+] to fall and hence an increased pH and a slight decrease in [HCO_3-]. The compensatory response involves reduced H^+ secretion, increased HCO_3- excretion and decreased HCO_3- reabsorption, thus restoring pH. Correction involves rectification of the underlying respiratory defect.

Metabolic acidosis

The causes of metabolic acidosis are:

- Ingestion of acids (H^+)
- Excess metabolic production of H^+ (e.g. lactate acidosis, diabetic ketoacidosis)

- Loss of HCO_3^- (e.g. severe diarrhoea, drainage from fistulae)
- Renal disease (failure to excrete H^+).

ABG results show a normal pCO_2 and decreased pH. There is an increase in [H^+]. Therefore, the following equation is shifted to the left:

$$CO_2 + H_2O \leftharpoons H_2CO_3 \leftharpoons H^+ + HCO_3^-$$

Consequently, [HCO_3^-] falls as it is used to 'mop up' the excess H^+ ions.

The decreased pH stimulates respiration to cause hyperventilation. This respiratory compensation decreases pCO_2 and returns the pH to normal, although HCO_3^- falls further. The fall in HCO_3^- hinders the compensatory response of the kidneys, which is to increase HCO_3^- reabsorption and produce titratable acid.

The anion gap represents the difference between plasma anions and cations and represents unaccounted anions (e.g. phosphates, ketones, lactate):

$$\text{Anion gap} = ([K^+] + [Na^+]) - ([Cl^-] + [HCO_3^-])$$

The normal range is 8–16 mmol/L. Changes in the anion gap help define the cause of a metabolic acidosis. Metabolic acidosis due to diarrhoea or renal tubular acidosis does not alter the anion gap. Acidosis caused by renal failure, diabetes or lactic acidosis increases the anion gap.

Clinical Note

A primary decrease in plasma bicarbonate and a slight reduction in pH indicate a metabolic acidosis. This may be caused by failure of the kidneys to excrete H^+ or reabsorb HCO_3. This may be caused by renal tubular acidosis types I, II and IV. It is important to note that the acidosis refers to the plasma pH, not that of the tubular fluid and that the urine can be alkaline. Alkali is usually administered to correct the acidosis.

Metabolic alkalosis

The causes of metabolic alkalosis are:

- Loss of acid (e.g. vomiting, diarrhoea)
- Ingestion of alkali (e.g. antacid ingestion)
- Depleted ECF (e.g. haemorrhage, burns, excess diuretic use, contraction alkalosis).

ABG results show a normal pCO_2 and an elevated pH because of a rise in plasma $[HCO_3^-]$. Therefore, the following equation is shifted to the right:

$$CO_2 + H_2O \leftrightharpoons H_2CO_3 \leftrightharpoons H^+ + HCO_3^- H^+ + OH^- \rightarrow H_2O$$

Consequently, $[HCO_3^-]$ is increased.

Respiratory compensation occurs. The increase in pH acts on chemoreceptors, which reduce the ventilatory rate and so increase pCO_2. The equation therefore shifts to the right and the pH returns to normal, but HCO_3^- increases further. This hinders correction.

Fig. 3.9 summarizes acid–base disturbances.

REGULATION OF CALCIUM AND PHOSPHATE

Calcium

Ca^{2+} is present mainly in bone but has an important extraskeletal function. The threshold potential of cell membranes of nerve and muscle for action potentials varies inversely with plasma calcium concentration. Thus it is important to keep calcium levels constant.

Calcium exists in two forms in the plasma:

1. Ionized Ca^{2+}, which is physiologically more important (normal concentration: 1.25 mmol/L)
2. Ca^{2+} bound to protein – mainly albumin (normal concentration: 1.25 mmol/L).

Ca^{2+} concentrations are:

- Total plasma Ca^{2+}: 2.2–2.6 mmol/L. Half is ionized (and physiologically more important) and half is bound to protein.
- Intracellular Ca^{2+}: 0.0001 mmol/L. It is important to maintain this low intracellular Ca^{2+} as it is involved in cell signaling pathways.

Calcium and phosphate homeostasis

Ca^{2+} and PO_4^{3-} precipitate to form insoluble calcium phosphate and their concentrations in the blood are close to the saturation point. Adding more of one of the ions results in the precipitation of some calcium phosphate thus some of the other ion is removed from

Fig. 3.9 Summary of acid–base disturbances and compensatory mechanisms.

Acid–base disturbance	PH	PCO_2	HCO_3^-	Clinical cause	Compensation
Respiratory acidosis	↓	↑	↑	Severe asthma; COPD	Metabolic (↑ HCO_3^-)
Respiratory alkalosis	↑	↓	↓	Hyperventilation	Metabolic (↓ HCO_3^-)
Metabolic acidosis	↓	Normal	↓	Diabetic ketoacidosis; chronic renal failure	Respiratory (↓ pCO_2)
Metabolic alkalosis	↑	Normal	↑	Vomiting	Respiratory (↑ pCO_2)

the solution. Hence, Ca^{2+} and PO_4^{3-} concentrations are inversely proportional.

$$[Ca^{2+}] \times [PO_4^{3-}] = constant$$

Therefore, a rise in Ca^{2+} leads to a decrease in PO_4^{3-} whereas a fall in Ca^{2+} stimulates an increase in PO_4^{3-} concentration, and vice versa.

Ca^{2+} and PO_4^{3-} enter the ECF via the intestine (diet) and bone stores. They leave the ECF via the kidneys (urine) and move into the bone.

Parathyroid hormone

PTH is a polypeptide secreted by the parathyroid gland when there is a fall in plasma Ca^{2+}. PO_4^{3-} also affects PTH release, both directly and secondary to changes in Ca^{2+} levels. Fig 3.10 illustrates mechanisms of Ca^{2+} and PO_4^{3-} homeostasis. Vitamin D can also affect PTH release because it alters sensitivity of the parathyroid gland to Ca^{2+}.

Vitamin D

Vitamin D refers to a group of closely related sterols obtained from the diet or by the action of ultraviolet light on certain provitamins. It is metabolized to 1,25-dihydroxycholecalciferol by the liver and kidney. This causes an increase in Ca^{2+} and PO_4^{3-} by:

- Enhancing intestinal absorption of Ca^{2+}
- Increasing Ca^{2+} release from bone
- Decreasing Ca^{2+} and PO_4^{3-} excretion.

Calcitonin

Calcitonin is a peptide produced by the parafollicular cells of the thyroid. It has the opposite effect to PTH, reducing Ca^{2+} release from bone and causing a decrease in ECF Ca^{2+} concentration.

Ca^{2+} transport by the kidney

Only ionized Ca^{2+} is filtered through the glomerulus (approximately 50% plasma Ca^{2+}). Reabsorption proceeds as follows:

- Proximal tubule: 70% is reabsorbed by diffusion, Ca^{2+}-activated ATPase and the Ca^{2+}/Na^+ counter-transport system
- Thick ascending loop of Henle: 20–25% is reabsorbed passively

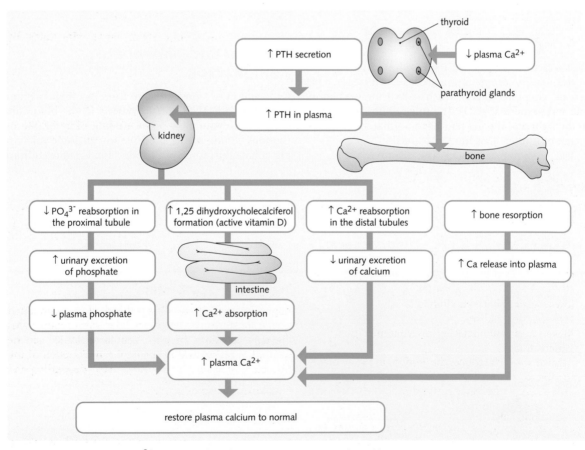

Fig. 3.10 Mechanisms of Ca^{2+} and phosphate homoeostasis. PTH, parathyroid hormone.

- Distal convoluted tubule: 5–10% is reabsorbed against an electrochemical gradient
- Collecting tubule: less than 0.5% is reabsorbed against an electrochemical gradient.

Phosphate

Phosphate (PO_4^{3-}) salts are essential for the structure of bones and teeth. Eighty per cent of the body's PO_4^{3-} content is in bone and 20% is in the intracellular fluid (ICF). It is filtered easily at the glomerulus; 80% is then reabsorbed in the proximal tubule and the remaining 20% is excreted in urine.

The kidneys play an important role in the regulation of PO_4^{3-}. Reabsorption of PO_4^{3-} occurs with Na^+ ions (two Na^+ for every PO_4^{3-} ion) at the apical membrane of the tubular cells. Any increase in plasma PO_4^{3-} concentration (>1.2 mmol/L) leads to an increase in the amount filtered and excreted, which is how plasma PO_4^{3-} levels are controlled. A fall in GFR will result in increased plasma PO_4^{3-} concentration. This hyperphosphataemia is a common cause of itching in CKD.

PO_4^{3-} is an important urinary buffer for H^+ and its excretion is influenced by:

- Parathyroid hormone (increases excretion)
- Vitamin D (decreases excretion)
- Acidosis (increases excretion)
- Glucocorticoids (increases excretion).

Clinical features and causes of Ca^{2+} disturbances

Hypocalcaemia

Decreased Ca^{2+} results in neuromuscular excitability leading to tetany with convulsions, hand and feet muscle cramps and cardiac arrhythmias.

Causes are:

- Chronic kidney disease, due to hyperphosphataemia (if PO_4^{3-} rises, Ca^{2+} must fall proportionally) and low levels of activated vitamin D
- Hypoparathyroidism
- Rickets and osteomalacia (low vitamin D)
- Pancreatitis
- Alkalosis, which reduces the amount of H^+ available to bind to protein, so more Ca^{2+} can bind to protein. This results in decreased ionized Ca^{2+}, although total Ca^{2+} remains the same.

Treatment is with oral or intravenous calcium and patients with chronic kidney disease will benefit from alfacalcidol, a vitamin D analogue.

Hypercalcaemia

Causes of hypercalcaemia are:

- Primary hyperparathyroidism
- Sudden acidosis, resulting in the release of bound calcium, which becomes ionized Ca^{2+}
- Increased intestinal absorption due to excess vitamin D or ingestion of calcium (milk–alkali syndrome)
- Bone destruction resulting in increased Ca^{2+} release from bone – usually caused by secondary deposits from malignancy or myeloma
- Production of humoral hypercalcaemic agents by tumours
- Granulomatous disease (sarcoid)
- Drugs, e.g. thiazides
- Tertiary hyperparathyroidism in chronic kidney disease
- Hypermagnesaemia.

Symptoms and signs of hypercalcaemia are:

- Polyuria
- Polydipsia.
- 'Bones' (bone pain and fractures)
- 'Stones' (renal calculi)
- 'Groans' (abdominal pain, vomiting and constipation)
- 'Moans' (depression or confusion).

Treatment is of the underlying cause, with fluids for rehydration and bisphosphonates.

Clinical Note

CKD results in hyperphosphataemia and hypocalcaemia with high parathyroid hormone and low activated vitamin D levels. This leads to renal osteodystrophy.

REGULATION OF POTASSIUM AND MAGNESIUM

Potassium

Transport of potassium

Approximately 70% of K^+ is reabsorbed in the proximal tubule, mostly by passive paracellular reabsorption across the tight junctions between tubular cells. K^+ can be secreted or reabsorbed in the nephron. Excretion of the filtered K^+ can vary from 1% to 110% depending on:

- Dietary intake of potassium
- Acid-base status
- Aldosterone levels.

K^+ reabsorption occurs mainly in the thick ascending loop of Henle by co-transport of $Na^+/K^+/Cl^-$ on the luminal membrane. Reabsorption of K^+ occurs in the distal tubule during severe dietary depletion of K^+.

Potassium (K^+) is the main intracellular cation. The intracellular and extracellular $[K^+]$ is very important in the function of excitable tissues (e.g. nerves and muscles) as it determines the resting potentials of these tissues. Therefore, a constant $[K^+]$ is critical for survival. Concentration is as follows:

- Total body K^+: 3–4 mmol/L
- Intracellular fluid (ICF) K^+: 98%; 150–160 mmol/L
- Extracellular fluid (ECF) K^+: 2%; 4–5 mmol/L.

K^+ transport by the kidney

K^+ is filtered freely in the glomerulus. The proximal tubule reabsorbs 80–90%:

- Passively
- Through tight junctions (paracellular movement)
- Via a concentration gradient.

Fig. 3.11 Potassium transport in the kidney.

In the distal tubule:

- K^+ reabsorption and leakage back are approximately equal in the early distal tubule
- The late distal tubule and collecting ducts secrete K^+ into the urinary filtrate (passively via an electrochemical gradient) according to the body's needs – increased cellular K^+ concentration results in increased secretion and vice versa.

Changes in the distal tubular lumen also influence the rate of K^+ secretion. Fig. 3.11 illustrates K^+ transport in the kidney.

ADH stimulates the secretion of K^+ by the collecting ducts by enhancing Na^+ reabsorption. Aldosterone increases K^+ secretion. Increased plasma K^+ concentration stimulates aldosterone production by the adrenal cortex, so plasma aldosterone concentration rises. This in turn increases K^+ secretion and therefore K^+ excretion.

Hypokalaemia

Causes of a decreased K^+ concentration are:

- Vomiting
- Diarrhoea
- Diuretics
- Excess insulin (e.g. Cushing's syndrome, steroids)
- Renal tubular acidosis.

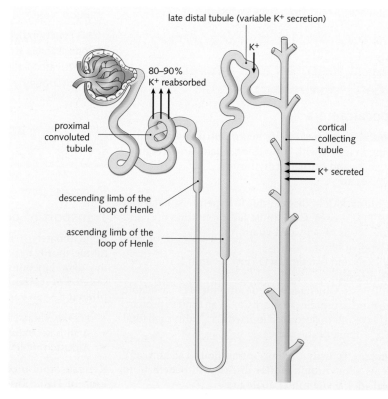

Hypokalaemia is asymptomatic until K^+ concentration falls below 2–2.5 mmol/L. The low K^+ concentration results in a decreased resting potential (more negative) so the nerve and muscle cells become hyperpolarized. This means that cells are less sensitive to depolarizing stimuli and therefore less excitable, so fewer action potentials are generated and paralysis ensues. Clinical effects of hypokalaemia are:

- Muscle weakness, cramps and tetany, which starts in the lower extremities and progresses upwards (death is usually by paralysis of respiratory muscles)
- Impaired liver conversion of glucose to glycogen
- Vasoconstriction and cardiac arrhythmias
- Impaired ADH action, causing thirst and polyuria and no concentration of urine
- Metabolic alkalosis due to an increase in intracellular H^+ concentration.

Treatment involves treating the underlying cause, and calculated oral or intravenous administration of potassium salt may be required.

Hyperkalaemia

Hyperkalaemia can result from:

- Reduced renal excretion: due to acute kidney injury or chronic kidney disease, mineralocorticoid deficiency (e.g. Addison's disease), potassium-sparing diuretics or renal tubular defects
- Increased plasma load: due to dietary changes or cellular tissue breakdown
- Transcellular shift of potassium out of cells: due to metabolic acidosis, insulin deficiency, exercise or drugs (e.g. digoxin)
- Pseudohyperkalaemia, an artefact: due to haemolysis during venepuncture or storage of the sample, a high white cell or high platelet count.

Clinical features

Very similarly to hypokalaemia, it may be asymptomatic or cause muscle weakness. Importantly it can cause cardiac arrhythmias by influencing myocardial excitability (Fig. 3.12).

Treatment
- Calcium gluconate: This does not alter the potassium concentration but Ca^{2+} stabilizes the myocardium, preventing arrhythmias
- Insulin: This acts to drive potassium into cells, thus lowers plasma $[K^+]$ but does not remove potassium from the body. It is given with glucose to avoid hypoglycaemia
- Salbutamol: This also drives potassium into cells when given nebulized or i.v. but should not be used in patients with ischaemic heart disease or arrhythmias

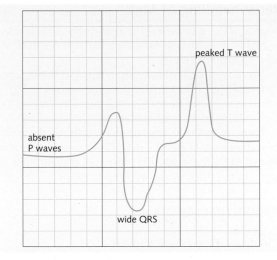

Fig. 3.12 ECG changes in hyperkalaemia. There are peaked T waves, absent P waves and broad QRS complexes. Eventually the pattern looks sinusoidal and can cause arrhythmias.

- Sodium bicarbonate: Correction of acidosis would also drive potassium into cells. Not used in patients at risk of fluid overload
- Calcium resonium: The removes K^+ by increasing its excretion from the bowels, given orally or by enema. This is the only way to remove K^+ from the body, apart from renal replacement therapy
- Renal replacement therapy: Dialysis or haemofiltration are used if medical therapies fail to correct hyperkalaemia.

Clinical Note

Emergency treatment of Hyperkalaemia > 6.5 mmol/L or ECG changes
- Continuous ECG monitoring
- 10 ml 10% calcium gluconate i.v.
- 15 units actrapid insulin $+ 50$ ml 50% glucose
- Continue with calcium resonium until $K^+ < 5.5$ mmol/L.

Magnesium

Magnesium (Mg^{2+}) is an intracellular cation that:

- Controls mitochondrial oxidative metabolism and so regulates energy production
- Is vital for protein synthesis
- Regulates K^+ and Ca^{2+} channels in cell membranes.

The plasma concentration of magnesium is 2.12–2.65 mmol/L; about 20% is protein bound.

Renal handling of Mg^{2+}

Ionized Mg^{2+} is filtered at the glomerulus. 15% is reabsorbed in the proximal tubule and 60% in the thick ascending loop of Henle.

The T_m for Mg^{2+} absorption is equal to the concentration of Mg^{2+} filtered. Therefore, an increase in Mg^{2+} results in increased filtering, which therefore exceeds the T_m, resulting in increased excretion.

There is intrinsic regulation by cells of the thick ascending loop of Henle – if Mg^{2+} decreases, cell transport of Mg^{2+} increases. PTH increases reabsorption of Mg^{2+} in the thick ascending loop of Henle.

Hypomagnesaemia

Causes are:

- Decreased intake
- Diarrhoea
- Absorption disorder including fat absorption defects
- Renal wasting – intrinsic (Bartter's syndrome), extrinsic (diuretics, e.g. thiazides).

Clinical features are non-specific. A fall in Mg^{2+} is followed by a decreased Ca^{2+}, but the mechanism for this is unknown.

Transport of other solutes in the tubules

Glucose

Normal plasma glucose concentration is 2.5–5.5 mmol/L. Usually, 0.2–0.5 mmol of glucose is filtered every minute. An increase in the plasma glucose concentration results in a proportional increase in the amount of glucose filtered. Virtually all filtered glucose is reabsorbed in the proximal tubule, unless the amount of filtered glucose exceeds the resorptive capacity of the cells. Glucose is transported into the proximal tubule cells by symport against its concentration gradient. It is driven by the energy released from the transport of Na^+ down its electrochemical gradient because the Na^+/K^+ ATPase pump on the basolateral membrane maintains a low Na^+ concentration and negative potential within the cell (Fig. 3.13). This is an example of secondary active transport. The transport ratio is:

- 1:1 Na^+: glucose in the pars convoluta
- 2:1 Na^+: glucose in the pars recta.

T_m is the maximum tubular resorptive capacity for a solute (i.e. the point of saturation for the carriers), and this value can be calculated for glucose. There is a limited number of Na^+/glucose carrier molecules, so glucose reabsorption is T_m limited. Fig. 3.14 shows that the lowest renal threshold of glucose is at a plasma glucose concentration of 10 mmol/L. At this level, filtered glucose will begin to be excreted in the urine (glycosuria). If the plasma glucose concentration increases further even those nephrons with highest resorptive capacity become saturated, and glucose is excreted. Urinary glucose increases in parallel with plasma glucose.

Glycosuria occurs if:

- The filtered load exceeds the renal threshold
- T_m for glucose is lower than normal.

Clinical Note

If plasma glucose rises above 10 mmol/L (as in diabetes), glycosuria will develop. However, glycosuria may also occur in non-diabetic people with normal blood sugar levels as a result of certain inherited renal tubule disorders. This is called renal glycosuria. Renal glycosuria also happens in pregnancy because the T_m for glucose falls, and glucose is excreted in the urine. A glucose tolerance test may be required to differentiate renal glycosuria from diabetes.

Amino acids

Amino acids are the basic unit of proteins and are absorbed constantly from the gut. The plasma concentration of amino acids is 2.5–3.5 mmol/L. They are small molecules that filter easily through the glomerulus, with most reabsorption occurring in the proximal tubule. The transport is a secondary active process (by symport with Na^+) and is driven by Na^+/K^+ ATPase, as with glucose. There are at least five different transport systems coupled with Na^+ and these are responsible for the movement of different types of amino acid residue. This is a T_m-limited process, so amino aciduria results if the reabsorption mechanism is saturated or if the reabsorption mechanism is defective (e.g. in Fanconi's syndrome).

Urea

Urea is the end-product of protein metabolism, which occurs in the liver. Urea is transported to the kidneys via the blood. It is a small molecule that is filtered freely at the glomerulus. The normal plasma concentration of urea is 2.5–7.5 mmol/L. Urea concentration increases in the filtrate as a result of Na^+, Cl^- and water reabsorption. This allows passive reabsorption of 40–50% of urea along its concentration gradient; 50–60% of the filtered urea is excreted in the urine. ADH increases the permeability of the inner medullary collecting ducts to urea. The distal tubule and the outer medullary ducts are impermeable to urea.

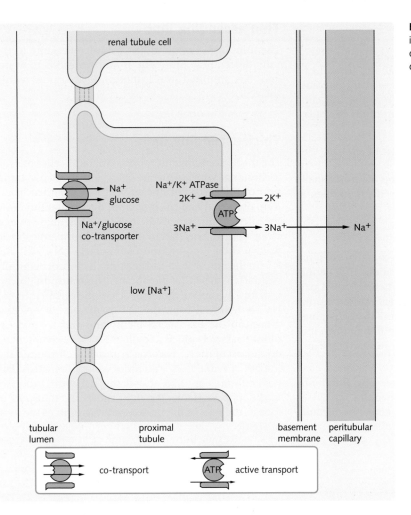

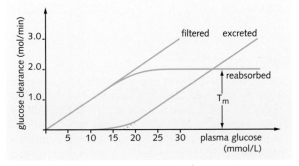

Fig. 3.14 Relation between plasma concentration, filtration, reabsorption and excretion of glucose (glomerular filtration rate = 100 mL/min). T_m is exceeded in nephrons with plasma glucose > 10 mmol/L and for all nephrons when plasma glucose > 20 mmol/L (nephron heterogeneity gives rise to 'splay' on the curve).

Sulphate

The normal plasma concentration of sulphate is 1–1.5 mmol/L. Sulphate reabsorption is T_m limited and this is an important mechanism in regulating its plasma concentration.

THE LOOP OF HENLE

Role of the loop of Henle

The loop of Henle reabsorbs 20% of the filtered Na^+ and 15% of tubular water. As filtrate flows through the loop of Henle, reabsorption of NaCl in the thick ascending limb produces a hypertonic interstitial fluid in the surrounding medulla. This creates a concentration gradient and water moves passively out of the thin descending limb.

The tubular fluid is isotonic to the plasma on entering the loop of Henle; however, by the time it leaves the loop it is hypotonic because ion reabsorption occurs within the loop. This mechanism allows urine to be concentrated, using the least amount of energy, because water is then reabsorbed passively from the collecting ducts into the hypertonic interstitium of the medulla.

Structure of the loop of Henle

The different components of the loop are functionally separate units, each with its own specific properties.

Thin descending limb

The thin descending limb is lined by thin, flat cells that have minimal cytoplasmic specialization. It is permeable to water, Na^+ and Cl^-. Water is reabsorbed passively down a concentration gradient caused by the hypertonic interstitium of the medulla. NaCl moves into the lumen and water moves out of the lumen into the interstitium, allowing the tubular fluid to come into equilibrium with the interstitium.

- The juxtamedullary nephrons have long, thin limbs that extend deep into the inner medulla
- The cortical nephrons only just enter the medulla and some are situated entirely in the cortex.

Thin ascending limb

The thin ascending limb has a similar structure to the thin descending limb but is impermeable to water and has minimal NaCl transport occurring within the cells.

Thick ascending limb

The thick ascending limb consists of large cells with mitochondria, which generate energy for the active transport of Na^+ (20% of filtered Na^+ is reabsorbed in the loop of Henle) and Cl^- ions from the tubular fluid into the interstitium. As a result, the filtrate becomes progressively diluted (this part of the tubule is impermeable to water). There is co-transport (symport) of Na^+, Cl^- and K^+ (in the ratio 1:2:1 – so the pump is electrochemically neutral) on the apical membrane. This transport process is driven by the Na^+ gradient across the cell membrane. Na^+ is removed from the cell by the Na^+/K^+ ATPase pump on the basolateral membrane and K^+ and Cl^- diffuse passively out as a result of Na^+ movement; however, most of the K^+ leaks back into the cell and tubular lumen. Overall, NaCl accumulates in the medullary interstitium. Fig. 3.15 shows the transport processes in the loop of Henle; the inset shows the transport of ions in the cells in the thick ascending limb of the loop of Henle.

Fig. 3.15 (A) Transport processes in the loop of Henle.

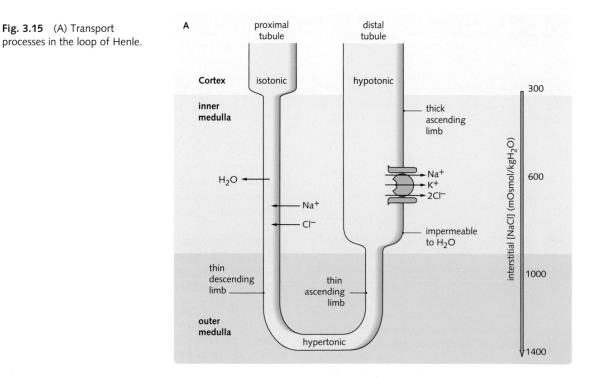

Continued

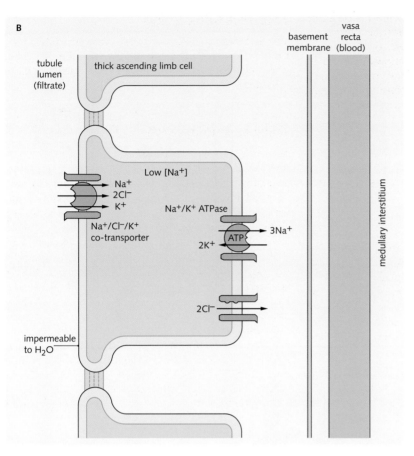

B

tubule lumen (filtrate)

thick ascending limb cell

basement membrane

vasa recta (blood)

medullary interstitium

Low [Na$^+$]

Na$^+$
2Cl$^-$
K$^+$

Na$^+$/Cl$^-$/K$^+$ co-transporter

Na$^+$/K$^+$ ATPase

ATP

3Na$^+$

2K$^+$

2Cl$^-$

impermeable to H$_2$O

Fig 3.15, cont'd (B) Transport of ions in the thick ascending limb.

Countercurrent multiplication

Any mechanism that will concentrate urine must be able to reabsorb water from the tubular fluid as it passes through the collecting ducts. The loop of Henle, which acts as a countercurrent multiplier, produces a hypertonic medulla by pooling NaCl in the interstitium, which favours the subsequent movement of water out of the collecting ducts (under the regulation of ADH). Each portion of the loop contributes to the effectiveness of this system.

The mechanism of the countercurrent multiplier is illustrated in Fig. 3.16. The thick, ascending limb can maintain a difference of 200 mOsmol/kg H$_2$O between the tubular fluid and the interstitium at any point along its length. The maximum osmolality of the interstitium is 1400 mOsmol/kg H$_2$O (normal plasma osmolality is 300 mOsmol/kg H$_2$O) at the tip of the loop. The fluid leaving the loop of Henle is hypotonic (100 mOsmol/kg H$_2$O).

Role of vasa recta and urea

The countercurrent mechanism requires an environment in which the waste products and water are cleared without disturbing the solutes that maintain the medullary hypertonicity. This exchange is provided by the vasa recta capillary system derived from the efferent arterioles of the longer juxtaglomerular nephrons. It does not require metabolic energy.

The capillaries have a hairpin arrangement surrounding the loop of Henle and are permeable to water and solutes. As the descending vessels pass through the medulla they absorb solutes such as Na$^+$, urea and Cl$^-$. Water moves along its osmotic gradient out of the capillaries. At the tip of the loop the capillary blood has the same osmolality as the interstitium, and an osmotic equilibrium is reached. The capillaries that ascend with the corresponding loop of Henle contain very viscous concentrated blood as a result of the earlier loss of water from the capillaries. A consequent increase in oncotic pressure because of the concentration of plasma proteins favours the movement of water back into the blood vessel from the interstitium. However, most of the NaCl is retained in the interstitium to maintain the hypertonic medullary environment.

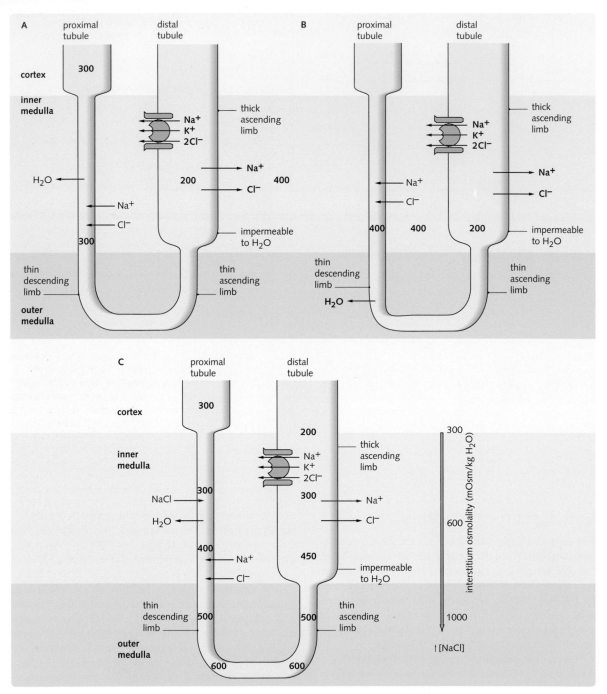

Fig. 3.16 (A) Active reabsorption occurs in the thick ascending limb, increasing the osmolality of the medulla (400 mOsmol/kg H$_2$O). The tubular fluid therefore decreases in osmolality (200 mOsmol/kg H$_2$O). (B) The increase in interstitial osmolality stimulates H$_2$O to leave the descending limb into the medulla. At the same time, increased interstitial osmolality results in passive diffusion of NaCl out of the medulla into the tubule until equilibrium is reached (400 mOsmol/kg H$_2$O). (C) The fluid in the tubule is progressively concentrated in descending the tubule as it comes into equilibrium with its surroundings (maximum value of 600 mOsmol/kg H$_2$O at the tip of the loop) and hence progressively diluted as it ascends the loop. This is all due to active NaCl reabsorption in the thick ascending limb (and some passive movement of NaCl in the ascending limb). Therefore a longitudinal gradient is set up, with greatest osmolality in the lower medulla and least in the cortex.

The collecting tubules pass through the cortex and medulla. They consist of two functionally different parts:

1. The cortical collecting ducts
2. The medullary (inner and outer) collecting ducts.

Both parts are impermeable to NaCl. The permeability to water and urea (only in the inner medullary collecting ducts) varies according to the presence of ADH. ADH increases the permeability to water and thus controls the concentration of the urine produced. ADH acts to increase water uptake in the cortical collecting tubules resulting in the production of a more concentrated urine.

The water reabsorbed in the medullary part of the collecting ducts is taken up by the vasa recta to prevent dilution of the medullary interstitium, which is crucial to the function of the distal nephron and the concentration of urine.

Although about 20% of the initial glomerular filtrate enters the distal nephron, only 5% enters the medullary

collecting ducts. This is mainly due to water reabsorption in the cortical tubules.

HINTS AND TIPS

The structure, location and function of the loop of Henle has a central role in the development of a hypertonic gradient in the medulla. This allows urine to be concentrated as it passes through the collecting tubules.

Fig. 3.17 shows the countercurrent exchanger and the collecting duct as it passes through the medulla.

Although urea is impermeable in the cortical collecting tubules, ADH affects the permeability of urea within the medullary cortical tubules. Urea, along with NaCl, helps maintain medullary hypertonicity as follows

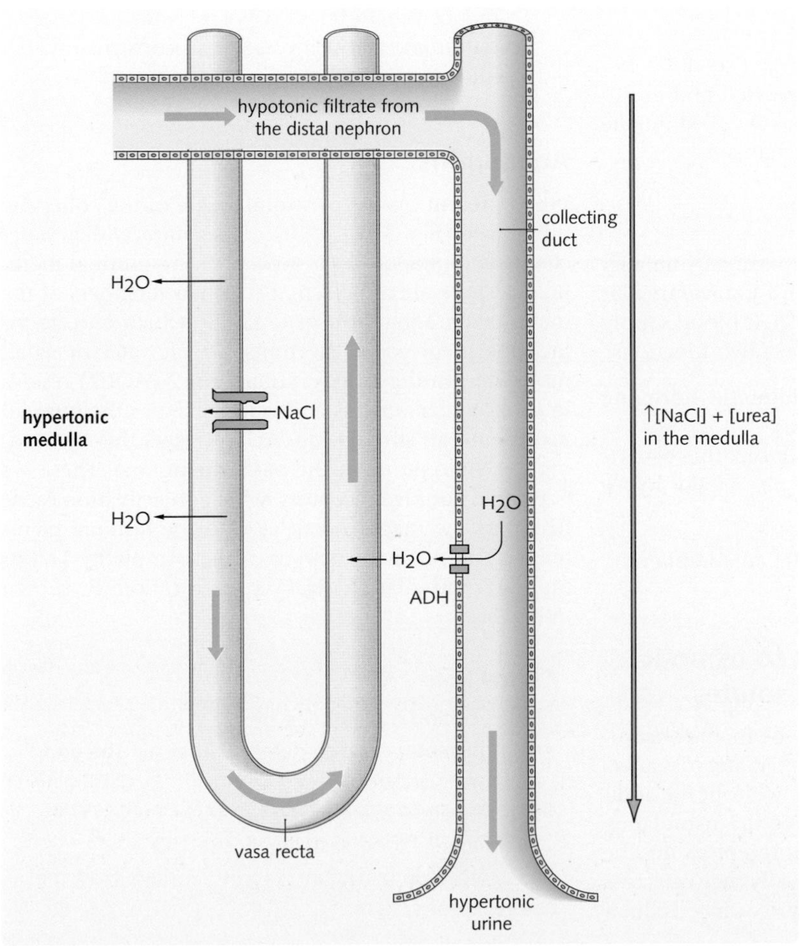

Fig. 3.17 Countercurrent exchanger as it passes through the medulla. The descending vessels of the vasa recta lose water as they pass through the hypertonic medulla. As a result of increasing oncotic pressure in the ascending vessels, water is reabsorbed passively back into the blood vessels from the interstitium as water uptake occurs in the collecting ducts under the influence of antidiuretic hormone (ADH). Because of this uptake of water by the vasa recta, the high osmolality of the medullary interstitium is maintained and this hypertonic environment allows continued concentration of the tubular fluid in the collecting duct.

- 50% of the filtered urea is reabsorbed in the proximal tubule with Na^+
- The tubular concentration of urea increases as it diffuses out of the medullary interstitium into the lumen down its concentration gradient
- The remaining urea becomes further concentrated within the tubular lumen as water and other solutes are reabsorbed into the cells of the distal tubule and the cortical collecting tubules, a process aided by the fact that these parts of the nephron are impermeable to urea
- The concentration of urea in the medullary collecting tubules is so high that it diffuses out of the lumen into the interstitium, thus increasing the concentration of urea in the medulla and recycling it. This occurs in the presence of ADH.

A high-protein diet increases the amount of urea in the blood for excretion as a result of increased metabolism. Consequently, there is more urea in the medullary interstitium, resulting in a higher urine osmolality.

Body fluid osmolality

Concepts of osmolality

The normal plasma osmolality (P_{osm}) is 285–295 mOsmol/kg H_2O. This is strictly regulated and an increase or decrease of 3 mOsmol/kg H_2O will stimulate the body's osmolality regulation mechanism.

Osmoreceptors

Osmoreceptors detect changes in the plasma osmolality and are located in the supraoptic and paraventricular areas of the anterior hypothalamus. Their blood supply is the internal carotid artery. They have two functions:

1. To regulate the release of antidiuretic hormone (ADH, also known as vasopressin)
2. To regulate thirst (this also depends on other osmoreceptors in the lateral preoptic area of the hypothalamus).

Fig. 3.18 illustrates the role of ADH in maintaining osmolality.

Sensitivity of osmoreceptors to osmotic changes caused by different solutes

Na^+ and other associated anions are the main constituents that determine plasma osmolality. Water loss alters the Na^+ concentration. Other solutes without the addition or loss of water can also change the osmolality. Not all solutes stimulate the osmoreceptors to the same degree – this depends on how easily they can cross the cell membrane (i.e. their ability to cause cellular dehydration).

Antidiuretic hormone (vasopressin)

Synthesis and storage

ADH is a peptide hormone synthesized in the supraoptic nucleus of the hypothalamus as a large precursor molecule. It is transported to the posterior pituitary gland, where its synthesis is completed and it is stored until release (Fig. 3.19).

Release

A rise in plasma osmolality triggers ADH release. Action potentials in the neurons from the hypothalamus (which contains ADH) depolarize the axon membrane, resulting in Ca^{2+} influx, fusion of secretory granules with the axon membrane and the release of ADH and neurophysin into the bloodstream.

Cellular actions

ADH has two functions:

1. To reduce water excretion (V_2 receptor-mediated)
2. To stimulate blood vessel vasoconstriction (V_1 receptor-mediated).

Aquaporins

When present on the peritubular side of the collecting tubule cell (Fig. 3.20), ADH causes intracellular water channels (aquaporins) to fuse with the luminal membrane. There are at present 11 known members of the mammalian aquaporin gene family which encode for proteins involved in the transport of water or small molecules. In the kidney, aquaporin 2 (AQP2) resides in intracellular vesicles and is trafficked to the luminal membrane on stimulation. ADH triggers this by binding to V_2 receptors on the basal membrane. These are G-protein-coupled receptors, which on activation cause fusion of the inactive vesicles with the luminal membrane. The relation between urine osmolality (mOsmol/kg) and plasma ADH concentration is shown in Fig. 3.21.

> **Clinical Note**
>
> ADH secretion is controlled by:
> - Osmoreceptors (which detect changes in the body fluid osmolarity)
> - Baroreceptors (which detect changes in blood volume, i.e. blood vessel wall 'stretch')
>
> The osmoreceptor system is more sensitive than the baroreceptor system.

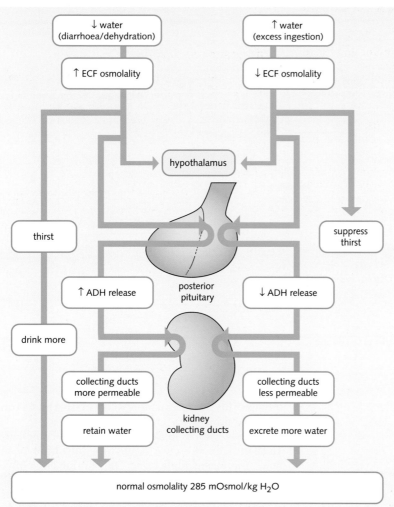

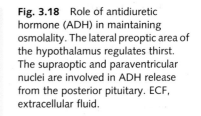

Fig. 3.18 Role of antidiuretic hormone (ADH) in maintaining osmolality. The lateral preoptic area of the hypothalamus regulates thirst. The supraoptic and paraventricular nuclei are involved in ADH release from the posterior pituitary. ECF, extracellular fluid.

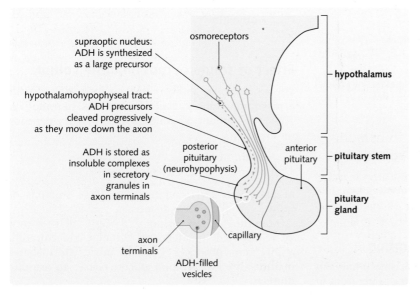

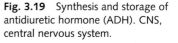

Fig. 3.19 Synthesis and storage of antidiuretic hormone (ADH). CNS, central nervous system.

Fig. 3.20 Actions of antidiuretic hormone (ADH) in the collecting tubule. AC, adenylate cyclase; cAMP, cyclic adenosine monophosphate; PKA, protein kinase; AQP2, aquaporin 2 water channel.

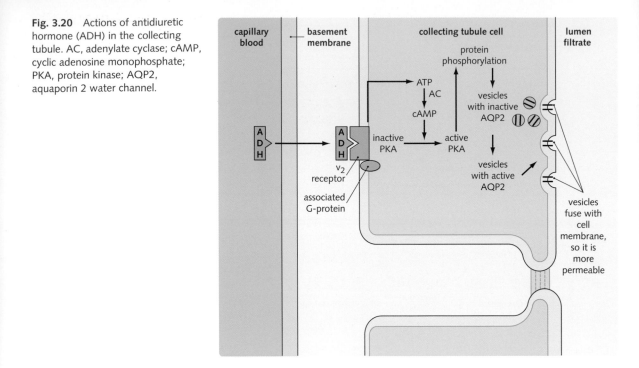

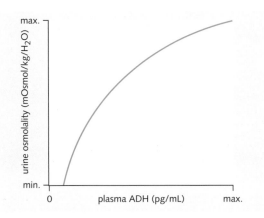

Fig. 3.21 Urine osmolality in relation to plasma antidiuretic hormone (ADH) concentration. (From Berne RM, Levy MN, 1996. Physiology, 3rd edn. Mosby Year Book.)

Drugs affecting ADH release

Drugs can:

- Increase ADH release (e.g. nicotine, ether, morphine, barbiturates)
- Inhibit ADH release (e.g. alcohol).

Water clearance and reabsorption

Dehydration leads to a rise in plasma osmolality. Thus, the kidneys reabsorb 'solute-free' water from the tubules. This produces a more dilute plasma and a concentrated urine.

Excessive water intake lowers plasma osmolality. Thus, the kidneys excrete 'solute-free' water from the tubules, producing dilute urine. Dilute urine has a lower osmolality than plasma, concentrated urine has a higher osmolality than plasma, isotonic urine has the same osmolality as plasma. The osmotic clearance (C_{osm}) (Fig. 3.22) is the rate at which osmotically active substances are cleared from the plasma. If urine is isotonic, C_{osm} = urine flow.

Effect of solute output on urine volume

The concentrating ability of the kidneys is limited, with a maximum urinary osmolality of 1400 mOsmol/kg. Thus, the amount of urine excreted per day depends on the:

- Amount of ADH
- Amount of solute excreted.

At maximum ADH concentration, large amounts of solutes can still cause a dieresis.

Mannitol is an osmotic diuretic that cannot be reabsorbed. It alters the kidney's concentrating ability and produces isotonic urine. In diabetes mellitus, the excess blood glucose causes an osmotic diuresis.

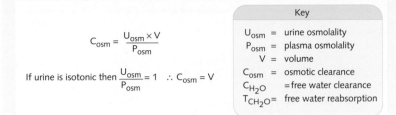

Fig. 3.22 Osmotic clearance. ADH, antidiuretic hormone.

$$C_{osm} = \frac{U_{osm} \times V}{P_{osm}}$$

If urine is isotonic then $\frac{U_{osm}}{P_{osm}} = 1$ ∴ $C_{osm} = V$

Key		
U_{osm}	=	urine osmolality
P_{osm}	=	plasma osmolality
V	=	volume
C_{osm}	=	osmotic clearance
C_{H_2O}	=	free water clearance
T_{CH_2O}	=	free water reabsorption

If urine osmolality < plasma osmolality, i.e. dilute urine production:

$$\frac{U_{osm}}{P_{osm}} < 1 \quad ∴ C_{osm} < V$$

The urine volume has additional free water and isotonic fluid

$$∴ V = C_{osm} + C_{H_2O}$$

Maximum C_{H_2O} = 12–15 mL/min (15–22 L/day)

If urine osmolality > plasma osmolality, i.e. concentrated urine produced:

$$\frac{U_{osm}}{P_{osm}} > 1 \quad ∴ C_{osm} > V$$

Here however, water is being excreted so

$$∴ V = C_{osm} - Tc_{H_2O}$$

Water is reabsorbed here so we can substitute (C_{H_2O}) for Tc_{H_2O}

C_{H_2O} and Tc_{H_2O} are quantitative ways of determining the ability of the kidney to excrete or conserve water

---

Clinical Note

In children younger than 5 years, bed wetting may be normal. However, repeated bedwetting in children over the age of 5 years may indicate a pathological cause and is called nocturnal enuresis. It occurs in about 10% of children aged 10, affecting boys more than girls. One cause is a reduction in circulating nocturnal antidiuretic hormone (ADH) levels. This may be managed by many methods, including the use of an ADH analogue called desmopressin, administered by a nasal spray.

Adrenal steroids and urinary dilution

Adrenal insufficiency leads to impaired water excretion (i.e. mineralocorticoid and/or glucocorticoid deficiency):

- Glucocorticoid deficiency can enhance water permeability of the collecting duct
- Glucocorticoid and mineralocorticoid deficiencies increase ADH levels, resulting in an inability to produce dilute urine. This is corrected by administering adrenal steroids.

DISORDERS OF OSMOLALITY

Hyponatraemia

In hyponatraemia, plasma [Na$^+$] is < 130 mmol/L and there is a decreased solute: water ratio in the extracellular fluid.

Causes

The causes of hyponatraemia are:

- Diuretics (mainly thiazides)
- Water overload or retention
- Increased antidiuretic hormone (ADH) secretion
- Increased plasma osmolarity (e.g. caused by mannitol, glucose)
- Increased protein or lipids (pseudohyponatraemia). Here, there is less sodium relative to the increase in protein or lipids, giving the impression of a low sodium.

The diagnostic approach to hyponatraemia is shown in Fig. 3.23.

Fig. 3.23 Diagnostic approach to hyponatraemia. ECF, extracellular fluid; SIADH, syndrome of inappropriate antidiuretic hormone secretion; TURP, transurethral resection of the prostate.

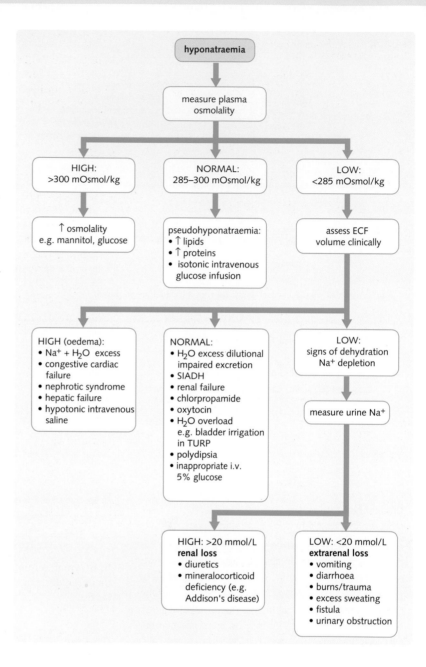

Syndrome of inappropriate ADH secretion (SIADH)

Occasionally ADH is secreted inappropriately by the pituitary or other areas in the body. Causes are given in Fig. 3.24. Signs and symptoms are:

- Hyponatraemia (<125 mmol/L) and low plasma osmolality (<260 mmol/L)
- Inappropriate urine osmolality: the urine concentration is higher than normal (i.e. not maximally diluted)

- Inappropriate Na^+ excretion: urinary $[Na^+]$ is greater than 20 mmol/L despite a decrease in plasma Na^+ concentration because the plasma volume is maintained by water retention (unless volume contracted or sodium restricted, which can decrease urinary Na^+).

The diagnosis should be considered in hyponatraemic patients in the absence of hypovolaemia, oedema, endocrine dysfunction, renal failure and drugs, all of which can impair water excretion.

Fig. 3.24 Causes of syndrome of inappropriate antidiuretic hormone secretion (SIADH)

Disorder	Example of finding
CNS disorders	Abscess, stroke, vasculitis (systemic lupus erythematosus)
Malignancy	Small cell carcinoma in lungs, duodenum, pancreas, prostate, ureter, adrenals
Lung diseases	Tuberculosis, pneumonia, abscess, aspergillosis
Drugs	Opiates, chlorpropamide, psychotropics, cytotoxics, narcotics, oxytocin
Metabolic diseases	Porphyria, hypothyroidism
Miscellaneous	Pain (postoperative), Guillain–Barré syndrome, trauma

Hypernatraemia

In hypernatraemia the serum sodium is >140 mmol/L and there is an increase in solute to water ratio in body fluids and increased serum osmolality (>300 mOsmol/kg).

Causes

The causes of hypernatraemia are:

- Osmotic diuresis (e.g. uncontrolled diabetes)
- Fluid loss without replacement (sweating, burns, vomiting)
- Diabetes insipidus (suspect if lots of dilute urine is produced)
- Incorrect intravenous fluid replacement (i.e. hypertonic fluids)
- Primary aldosteronism.

A diagnostic algorithm is given in Fig. 3.25.

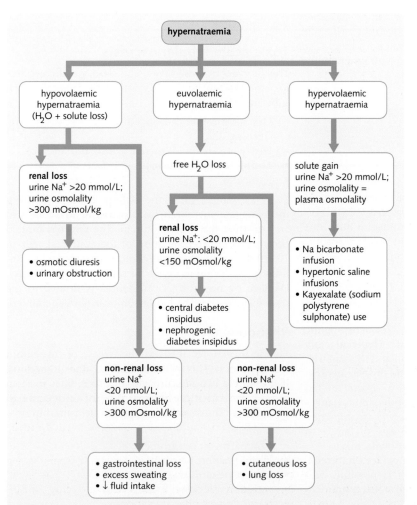

Fig. 3.25 Diagnostic approach to hypernatraemia.

Diabetes insipidus

This is the inability to reabsorb water from the distal part of the nephron, due to the failure of secretion or action of ADH. Symptoms are:

- Polyuria
- Polydipsia
- Low urine osmolality, i.e. dilute urine.

The causes of diabetes insipidus are:

- Neurogenic/central: impaired ADH synthesis or secretion by the hypothalamus, which might be congenital, caused by hypothalamic damage or due to pituitary tumours. It can be treated by administering ADH
- Nephrogenic: failure of the kidneys to respond to circulating ADH, which could be caused by mutations in the gene coding for V_2 receptors, chronic pyelonephritis, polycystic kidneys or drugs such as lithium. Plasma ADH levels are normal. There is no current treatment to correct the deficit.

Diabetes insipidus can be mistaken for psychogenic polydipsia, in which large volumes of dilute urine are produced secondary to compulsive water drinking. This causes a decrease in the urine-concentrating ability because of loss of medullary tonicity.

DISEASES OF THE TUBULES AND INTERSTITIUM

Overview

The tubules and interstitium are affected by several diseases. Typically, tubules become obstructed (this reduces glomerular filtration) or their transport functions become impaired (reduces water and solute reabsorption). Damage can be acute or chronic.

Acute tubular necrosis

Acute tubular necrosis (ATN) is the result of acute tubular cell damage by ischaemia or toxins. It can be oliguric (<400 mL/day urine) or non-oliguric. Hyperkalaemia can develop as a result of K^+ retention and this can trigger cardiac arrhythmias, which can be life-threatening. Uraemia develops because there is a significant fall in GFR – this could be due to haemodynamic changes and intratubular obstruction. Recovery is accompanied by a diuretic phase that occurs because of failure to concentrate urine (this can cause hypokalaemia).

ATN is a cause of acute kidney injury (see Chapter 7). Mortality is high but full recovery is possible with prompt treatment – fluid and electrolyte therapy and dialysis if necessary.

The tubular cells are capable of regenerating rapidly to allow complete recovery.

Ischaemic acute tubular necrosis

This is caused by hypotension and hypovolaemic shock following trauma, infections, burns or haemorrhage. There is a rapid fall in blood pressure, which causes hypoperfusion of the peritubular capillaries with consequent tubular necrosis along the entire length of the nephron. The kidneys appear pale and swollen. Histological examination reveals:

- Infiltration of inflammatory cells and the tubular cells
- Flattened and vacuolated tubular cells
- Interstitial oedema
- Cellular debris and protein casts in the distal tubule and the collecting ducts.

Non-steroidal anti-inflammatory drugs (NSAIDs) can increase the risk of ATN following other renal insults by preventing the synthesis of prostaglandins (PGs). PGs are vasodilators, which protect the kidney from ischaemic injury by dilating blood vessels and increasing blood flow.

Toxic acute tubular necrosis

This disorder is caused by agents with specific nephrotoxic activity causing damage to the epithelial cells. Such substances include:

- Organic solvents: carbon tetrachloride (CCl_4) in dry-cleaning fluid
- Heavy metals (gold, mercury, lead and arsenic)
- Antibiotics (gentamicin)
- Pesticides.

These substances cause the cells to come away from the basement membrane and consequently collect in and obstruct the tubular lumen. The effect is limited because there is regeneration of the epithelial cells in 10–20 days, which permits clinical recovery and is confirmed by the presence of mitotic figures on biopsy. Damage by nephrotoxic substances is limited to the proximal tubules. The kidneys appear swollen and red.

Rhabdomyolysis

Muscle breakdown leads to the release of myoglobin into the blood. This is filtered freely by the glomerulus. If the filtrate is acidic myoglobin precipitates to form casts which block the normal flow of urine through the tubules. The muscle damage can be caused by:

- Trauma
- Compartment syndrome
- Drugs (statins, heroin)
- Electrolyte abnormalities
- Infections (legionella, influenza)
- Neuroleptic malignant syndrome.

Investigations will reveal a very high creatine kinase (> 10 000) and hyperkalaemia from release from muscle cells. The urine will be dark and give a false positive for blood on a dipstick test.

Treatment involves stopping the damage to muscle tissue if possible. Intravenous fluids are given to promote high urine production alongside alkalinisation of the urine with sodium bicarbonate to help to decrease the precipitation of myoglobin in the tubules.

Tubulointerstitial nephritis

Pyelonephritis

This is a bacterial infection of the kidney and results in inflammation and damage to the renal calyces, parenchyma and pelvis. It can be acute or chronic.

Acute pyelonephritis

This occurs because of infection in the kidney and is spread via two routes:

1. Ascending infection: bacteria from the gut enter the kidney from the lower urinary tract if there is an incompetent vesicoureteric valve. This permits vesicoureteric reflux (VUR) and results in ascending transmission of infection
2. Haematogenous spread: seen in patients with septicaemia or infective endocarditis. The pathogens include fungi, bacteria (staphylococci and *Escherichia coli*) and viruses. The kidney is often affected in septicaemic diseases because of its large blood supply.

The predisposing factors of acute pyelonephritis are:

- Urinary tract obstruction (congenital and acquired)
- VUR
- Instrumentation of the urinary tract
- Sexual intercourse
- Diabetes mellitus
- Immunosuppression (human immunodeficiency virus infection, lymphoma and transplants).

Patients present with general malaise, fever, loin pain, tenderness and often rigors with or without symptoms of lower UTI. Infection spreads into the renal pelvis and papillae and causes abscess formation throughout the cortex and medulla.

With retrograde ureteric spread the kidney characteristically contains areas of wedge-shaped suppuration especially at the upper and lower poles. In septicaemia there is haematogenous seeding within the kidney and minute abscesses are distributed randomly in the cortex. On histological examination there is:

- Polymorphic infiltration of the tubules
- Interstitial oedema
- Focal inflammation.

Uncomplicated cases resolve with antibiotic treatment and high fluid intake. The important complications of acute pyelonephritis are:

- Renal papillary necrosis
- Perinephric abscesses
- Pyonephrosis (obstruction of the pelvicalyceal system)
- Chronic pyelonephritis
- Fibrosis and scarring.

Chronic pyelonephritis

This condition is characterized by long-standing parenchymal scarring, which develops from tubulointerstitial inflammation. It is the end-result of various pathological processes. There are two main types:

1. Obstructive: chronic obstruction (stones, tumours or congenital abnormalities) prevents pelvicalyceal drainage and increases the risk of renal infection. Chronic pyelonephritis develops because of recurrent infection
2. Reflux nephropathy: this is the most common cause of chronic pyelonephritis. It is associated with VUR, which is congenital. The organisms enter the ascending portion of the ureter with refluxed urine as the valvular orifice is held open on contraction of the bladder during micturition. Reflux results from the abnormal angle at which the ureter enters the bladder wall (Fig. 3.26).

The disease process usually begins in childhood and has a silent, insidious onset. Reflux of urine into the renal pelvis occurs during micturition and this increases the pressure in the major calyces. The high intrapelvic pressure forces urine into the collecting ducts with intraparenchymal reflux further distorting the internal structure. This is most predominant at the poles of the kidney and results in deep irregular scars on the cortical surface. The tubulointerstitial inflammation heals with the formation of corticomedullary scars that overlie the deformed and dilated calyces, which are characteristic of chronic pyelonephritis (Fig. 3.27).

On histological examination there is interstitial fibrosis and dilated tubules containing eosinophilic casts; 10–20% of patients requiring dialysis have chronic pyelonephritis.

Ultrasonography is used to diagnose chronic pyelonephritis and may show distortion of the calyceal system and contraction of the kidney because of cortical scarring. Intravenous pyelography may be more sensitive but requires exposure to X-rays which should be avoided, especially in children.

Fig. 3.26 Normal and refluxing (abnormal) junction.

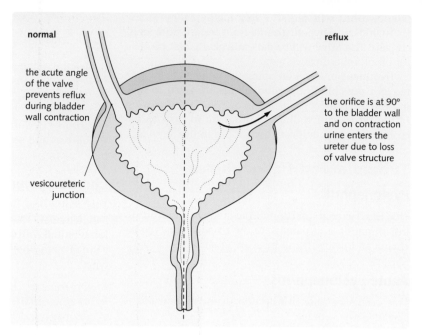

Fig. 3.27 Differences between (A) acute and (B) chronic pyelonephritis.

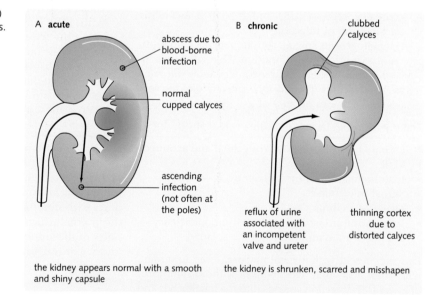

Toxin- and drug-induced tubulointerstitial nephritis

Heavy metals (mercury, gold, lead) and drugs (ampicillin, rifampicin, NSAIDs) can cause T-cell-mediated inflammation in the interstitium. This reaction usually occurs 2–40 days after exposure to the toxin. Clinical features include fever, skin rash, haematuria, proteinuria and ARF. Withdrawal of the causative agent leads to recovery.

On histological examination there is interstitial oedema and tubular degeneration with eosinophil infiltration. In chronic analgesic abuse with phenacetin, and to a lesser extent aspirin, PG synthesis is inhibited, causing ischaemia (as described on p. 50 for ischaemic ATN). This causes papillary necrosis and a secondary tubulonephritis (analgesic nephropathy). It is associated with an increased risk of developing transitional cell carcinomas with chronic analgesic abuse.

Clinical Note

Chronic analgesic misuse inhibits PG synthesis, causing ischaemia. The resultant papillary necrosis can be diagnosed in X-rays. It is seen in analgesic nephropathy, diabetes, sickle-cell disease and urinary tract obstruction.

Acute urate nephropathy

If there is an increased blood urate concentration, urate crystals are precipitated in the acidic environment of the collecting ducts, causing inflammatory obstruction and dilatation of the tubules. This is called acute urate nephropathy and causes acute kidney injury. A typical cause is tumour lysis syndrome. This involves rapid cell turnover in those patients with haematological or lymphatic malignancy who are receiving chemotherapy. There is excess cell breakdown and release of nucleic acids, which results in acute urate nephropathy and presents as Acute Kidney Injury.

HINTS AND TIPS

Chronic kidney disease can cause gout through reduced excretion of uric acid. However, chronic hyperuricaemia is now considered not to cause chronic nephropathy.

Hypercalcaemia and nephrocalcinosis

A persistently high blood Ca^{2+} level causes Ca^{2+} deposition in the kidneys. The hypercalcaemia can be due to:

- Primary hyperparathyroidism
- Multiple myeloma
- Increased vitamin D activity
- Bone metastases.

Renal insufficiency occurs in these patients because of stones (nephrolithiasis) or focal calcification in the renal parenchyma (nephrocalcinosis).

In nephrocalcinosis the Ca^{2+} accumulates in the tubular cells and the basement membrane, resulting in interstitial fibrosis and inflammation. Hypercalcaemia also causes a renal concentrating defect, which leads to polyuria, nocturia and dehydration.

Multiple myeloma

Approximately 50% of patients with multiple myeloma develop renal insufficiency, which can cause AKI or CKD. Histological changes include:

- Bence Jones proteins (light chains) enter the urine and these are toxic to the tubular epithelial cells. They combine with Tamm-Horsfall protein to precipitate as casts in the tubules, causing inflammation and obstruction to the tubular cells
- Amyloid lambda (λ) or kappa (κ) light-chain fragments (paraproteins) are deposited in the renal blood vessels, glomeruli and tubules
- Urate deposition (discussed above)
- Hypercalcaemia (discussed above).

Body fluid volume ④

By the end of the chapter you should be able to:
- Name the fluid compartments of the body and state their volume in a 70-kg male
- Explain the importance of sodium in the control of body fluid volume
- State where in the nephron most Na^+ and water are reabsorbed and state the mechanism
- Describe in detail the renin–angiotensin–aldosterone system and state the actions of angiotensin II
- Explain the renal responses to cardiac failure, liver failure and hypotension
- List six causes of hypertension and outline its management
- Understand the differences between the classes of diuretics and state which are considered the most powerful
- List the side effects of thiazide diuretics
- Describe the mechanism of action of potassium-sparing diuretics
- Understand the effects of ACE inhibitors in renal artery stenosis

CONTROL OF BODY FLUID VOLUME

Basic concepts

Body fluids

Body fluids are divided into:

- Intracellular fluid (ICF), the fluid within cells
- Extracellular fluid (ECF).

ECF is divided into:

- Plasma – ECF within the vascular system, i.e. the non-cellular component of blood
- Interstitial fluid (ISF) – ECF outside the vascular system (and separated from plasma by the capillary endothelium)
- Transcellular fluid (TCF) – ECF (e.g. synovial fluid, aqueous and vitreous humour, cerebrospinal fluid) separated from plasma by the capillary endothelium and an additional epithelial layer that has specialized functions (Fig. 4.1).

Water is a major component of the human body. Approximately 63% of an adult male and 52% of an adult female is water (i.e. 45 L in a 70-kg male, 36 L in a 70-kg female). This difference is due to the fact that females have a higher proportion of body fat, which has a low water content. One-third of total body water (TBW) is ECF (about 15 L in a 70-kg male) and two-thirds is ICF (about 30 L in a 70-kg male).

The volume of fluid that perfuses tissues is the effective circulating volume; this needs to be kept constant.

Sodium balance

Na^+ is the major cation in the extracellular fluid with a normal concentration of 135–145 mmol/L. It therefore controls 90% of body fluid osmolality. As discussed in the previous chapter, osmolality of the plasma is carefully controlled by the loop of Henle and collecting duct. Thus, changes in the amount of Na^+ in the ECF actually lead to changes in the ECF volume. For example, a rise in ECF Na^+ results in increased osmolality, which leads to water retention and thirst (increased drinking of water). This increases ECF volume and normalizes osmolality.

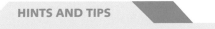

HINTS AND TIPS

The kidneys regulate the amount of Na^+ they reabsorb thus, alongside the mechanism regulating osmolality, they also control ECF volume.

Handling of sodium by the kidney

The concentration of Na^+ in the Bowman's capsule is equal to the plasma level because Na^+ is freely filtered. Virtually all the Na^+ that is filtered into the nephron is

Fig. 4.1 Fluid compartments of the body.

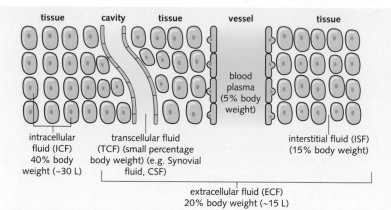

Fig. 4.2 Na$^+$ transport along the nephron.

Part of nephron	Percentage of filtered Na$^+$ reabsorbed	Method of entry into the cell	Regulatory hormones
Proximal tubule	65-70	Na$^+$ co-transport, paracellular	Angiotensin II
Loop of Henele	20-25	Na$^+$ /Cl$^-$ /K$^+$ pump (1:2:1)	Aldosterone
Early distal tubule	5	Na$^+$ /Cl$^-$ symport	Aldosterone
Late distal tubule and collecting ducts	5	Na$^+$ channels	Aldosterone, arial natriuretic peptide

reabsorbed back into the circulation, with only 1% or less of the filtered Na$^+$ being excreted in the urine (Fig. 4.2).

Transport of sodium in the proximal tubule

A lot of Na$^+$ is reabsorbed in the early proximal tubule but, as the cell junctions are leaky, the concentration gradient between the filtrate and the intercellular plasma is limited. Less reabsorption occurs in the late proximal tubule, but the cell junctions are tight so a better concentration gradient is established. The primary transporter Na$^+$/K$^+$ ATPase (Na$^+$ pump) on the basolateral membrane actively transports Na$^+$ out of the cell into the lateral intercellular spaces between adjacent cells (Fig. 4.3).

This movement of Na$^+$ out of the cell maintains a very low concentration of Na$^+$ within the proximal tubule cells. This drives Na$^+$ ions to move along their concentration gradients into the cells from the tubular fluid via carrier molecules on the apical membrane. In the early proximal tubule, movement of other substances, e.g. glucose, amino acids and PO$_4$$^{3-}$, is coupled with Na$^+$ transport in and out of tubule cells (discussed in the previous chapter).

The fluid leaving the proximal tubule is isosmotic because both ions and water move out of the filtrate together, i.e. it has no concentrating capacity.

The distal tubule and loop of Henle handling sodium

The complicated mechanism by which the loop of Henle handles sodium is dealt with in the previous chapter. This is mainly to create a concentration gradient to allow control of osmolality.

The distal convoluted tubule reabsorbs only around 10% of the filtered Na$^+$ but this is amount is adjustable and important in the control of body fluid volume. Sodium leaves the basolateral side through the Na$^+$/K$^+$ ATPase and enters the cell from the lumen through a Na$^+$/Cl$^-$ co-transporter, down its concentration gradient.

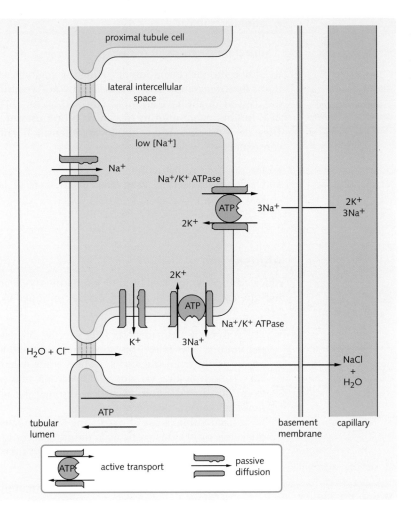

Fig. 4.3 Na^+ transport processes in the proximal tubule. Sodium entry into the cell is driven by its concentration gradient set up by the Na^+/K^+ ATPase pump found on the basal membrane.

Renin–angiotensin–aldosterone system

The renin–angiotensin–aldosterone system (Fig. 4.4) maintains Na^+ balance.

Renin

Renin is an enzyme that is synthesized and stored in the JGA in the kidneys. A fall in plasma Na^+ leads to a fall in ECF volume, causing the release of renin by:

- Increased sympathetic innervation: a fall in ECF volume results in a fall in blood pressure. This is detected by baroreceptors in carotid arteries and causes increased sympathetic activity. Granular cells of the JGA are innervated by the sympathetic system, so an increase in sympathetic activity leads to an increase in renin release. The process is mediated by ß-adrenergic receptors

- The wall tension in afferent arterioles falls: decreased ECF volume reduces blood pressure, which in turn decreases perfusion pressure to the kidneys. Changes in the blood pressure decrease wall tension at granular cells, which stimulates renin release
- Decreased Na^+ to the macula densa: if less NaCl reaches the macula densa, the macula densa is stimulated to secrete the prostaglandin PGI_2. This acts on the granular cells to cause renin release.

Conversion of angiotensinogen to angiotensin

Renin acts on angiotensinogen (α_2-globulin), which splits off angiotensin I (a decapeptide). Angiotensin-converting enzyme (ACE) in the lungs then removes two amino acids to produce angiotensin II (an octapeptide). Angiotensin II:

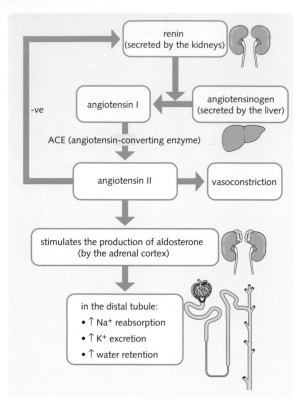

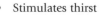

Fig. 4.4 The renin–aniotensin–aldosterone system. –ve, negative feedback.

- Stimulates the zona glomerulosa of the adrenal cortex to release aldosterone
- Directly vasoconstricts arterioles within the kidney (efferent > afferent)
- Directly increases Na^+ reabsorption from the proximal tubule
- Releases ADH

Fig. 4.5 Factors causing aldosterone release and the effects of aldosterone. ECF, extracellular fluid.

- Stimulates thirst
- Provides negative feedback to the JGA cells, and therefore affects renin release.

In addition to the generation of circulating angiotensin II, the local generation of angiotensin II by ACE (within the tissues) might have an important pathogenic role. ACE inhibitors are used to treat high blood pressure. They decrease the production of angiotensin II and consequently:

- Decrease vasoconstriction
- Decrease aldosterone (and prevent an increase in ECF volume).

Aldosterone

Aldosterone is synthesized by zona glomerulosa cells in the adrenal cortex. Its release (Fig. 4.5) is controlled by:

- Angiotensin II
- ECF volume: if circulating Na^+ falls, effective circulating volume also falls. This stimulates aldosterone release via the renin–angiotensin–aldosterone system
- Na^+ concentration: via direct aldosterone release from the adrenal cortex, as well as through the renin–angiotensin–aldosterone system
- K^+ concentration: a rise in circulating K^+ stimulates direct release of aldosterone from the adrenal cortex. This returns K^+ to normal by increasing distal tubular secretion of K^+.

Aldosterone primarily regulates sodium concentration. It acts within cells to:

- Promote Na^+ reabsorption in the kidney, colon, gastric glands and sweat and salivary gland ducts
- Promote K^+ and H^+ secretion by the kidney.

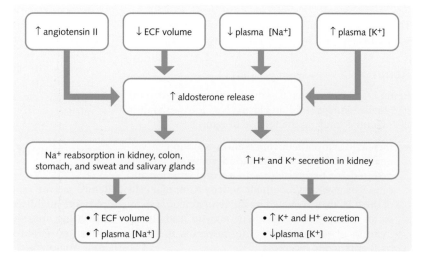

Clinical Note

Adrenal insufficiency is a condition where the adrenal glands fail to secrete the required hormone levels. It normally has a non-specific presentation unless the patient is having an acute adrenal crisis, which is typically life-threatening. On investigation, the patient may have abnormally high potassium levels (hyperkalaemia) and low sodium levels (hyponatraemia). These findings result from reduced aldosterone secretion and resultant renal Na^+ wasting and reduced K^+ excretion.

Other factors affecting Na^+ reabsorption

Starling's forces in the proximal tubule

The amount of Na^+ and water reabsorbed into the peritubular capillaries from the proximal tubule depends on the rate and amount of uptake from the lateral intercellular spaces into the capillaries.

Changes in the body fluid volume alter plasma hydrostatic and oncotic pressure, for example, increased NaCl intake is mirrored by a rise in ECF volume. This in turn increases hydrostatic pressure and decreases oncotic pressure, so NaCl and water reabsorption by the proximal tubule cells decreases.

Sympathetic drive from the renal nerves

The arterial baroreceptors regulate renal sympathetic nerve activity, for example, a fall in ECF volume decreases blood pressure, which is sensed by baroreceptors, and results in an increase in sympathetic activity. This stimulates Na^+ retention and an increase in peripheral resistance, thus restoring ECF volume and blood pressure.

A rise in sympathetic nerve activity to the kidney stimulates renin release either directly or as a result of renal vasoconstriction (this activates the JGA) (Fig. 4.6). Catecholamines from sympathetic nerve endings also stimulate Na^+ reabsorption by the proximal tubule, but it is unclear if this is a direct effect or secondary to altered peritubular forces.

Prostaglandins

A decrease in the effective circulating volume stimulates cortical prostaglandin (PG) synthesis. In the kidney, PG synthesis occurs in the:

- Cortex (arterioles and glomeruli)
- Medullary interstitial cells
- Collecting duct epithelial cells.

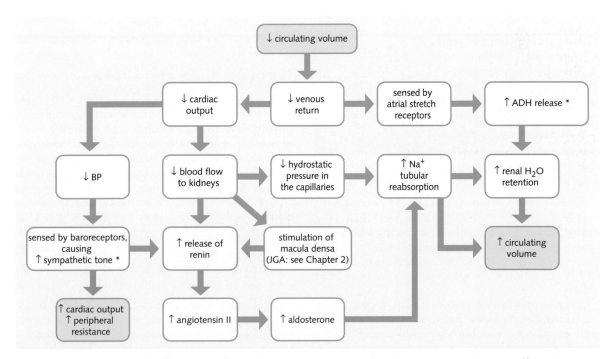

Fig. 4.6 Regulation of body fluid. JGA, Juxtaglomerular apparatus. Asterix (*) denotes ADH secretion is increased by an increase in sympathetic tone.

Several prostaglandins exist: PGE_2 (medullary), PGI_2 (cortical), $PGF_{2\alpha}$, PGD_2 and thromboxane A_2 (TXA_2). The main functions of each are as follows:

- PGE_2, PGI_2: vasodilators, preventing excessive vaso-constriction
- PGI_2 (prostacyclin): renin release
- PGE_2 (medullary): promotes water (diuretic) and sodium (natriuretic) excretion within the collecting tubules and thus overrides the antidiuretic action of ADH. PGE_2 protects the medullary tubule cells from excessive hypoxia when the ECF volume decreases
- TXA_2: a vasoconstrictor, which is synthesized after repeated kidney damage (e.g. ureteral obstruction). It reduces the amount of blood available for filtration by a poorly functioning kidney.

Atrial natriuretic peptide (ANP)

ANP is a peptide produced by cardiac atrial cells in response to an increase in ECF volume. It is found in the atrial cells and released into the plasma. ANP binds to specific cell surface receptors, resulting in increased cyclic guanosine monosulphate (cGMP). ANP acts to:

- Inhibit Na^+/K^+ ATPase and close Na^+ channels of the collecting ducts, reducing Na^+ reabsorption. Na^+ reabsorption is also reduced in the proximal tubules. Thus, Na^+ and water excretion by the kidney is increased
- Vasodilate afferent arterioles, thereby increasing GFR
- Inhibit aldosterone secretion
- Inhibit ADH release
- Decrease renin release.

RENAL RESPONSES TO SYSTEMIC DISORDERS

Congestive cardiac failure

Congestive cardiac failure (CCF) occurs when the heart muscle pump cannot cope with its work load. The cardiac output falls and fails to perfuse the tissues adequately. Hypoperfusion of the tissues results in sodium and water retention by the kidneys, leading to oedema. CCF is a common end result of all types of severe heart disease.

Renal hypoperfusion following a fall in cardiac output is sensed by the kidney as hypovolaemia resulting in compensation by retaining NaCl and water to increase the circulating volume (Fig. 4.7). As the kidney attempts to increase the circulating fluid volume, peripheral oedema develops. This increase in pulmonary venous pressure, results in fluid transudation from the capillaries in the lungs and in pulmonary oedema.

Treatment and management

Management involves reducing the fluid load within the body and thereby decreasing the workload of the heart.

- Diuretics: produce symptomatic relief from pulmonary oedema
- ACE inhibitors: act as vasodilators (by reducing the synthesis of angiotensin II) and as diuretics (by decreasing aldosterone synthesis)
- Nitrates: produce venodilation, which decreases preload
- Vasodilators (e.g. hydralazine): these reduce afterload.

Prognosis depends on the overall clinical picture, and the extent of cardiovascular disease. For further information see *Crash course: Cardiovascular system*.

Clinical Note

CCF can be caused by:
- Pump failure (low-output heart failure)
- Increased demand (high-output heart failure).

A normal heart can fail under high loads, but an abnormal heart will fail under normal loads.

The kidney tries to increase fluid volume, leading to peripheral oedema, and eventually pulmonary oedema.

Hypovolaemia and shock

Shock is a medical emergency in which the vital organs are inadequately perfused. As the amount of oxygen and nutrients delivered to the cells is inadequate, the resulting hypoxic state within the cells leads to anaerobic metabolism and there is inefficient clearance of the metabolites, which build up in the cell. Hypovolaemia and mild shock cause tiredness, dizziness and a feeling of thirst. A severe decrease in the circulating volume stimulates sympathetic activity to maintain the blood pressure by:

- Tachycardia
- Peripheral vasoconstriction
- Increase in myocardial contractility.

Vasodilation occurs in the vital organs (heart, lungs, brain) to maintain blood supply, but this is at the expense of perfusion to other organs. If there is inadequate compensation, tissue hypoxia and necrosis can occur in vulnerable organs (e.g. acute tubular necrosis in the kidneys).

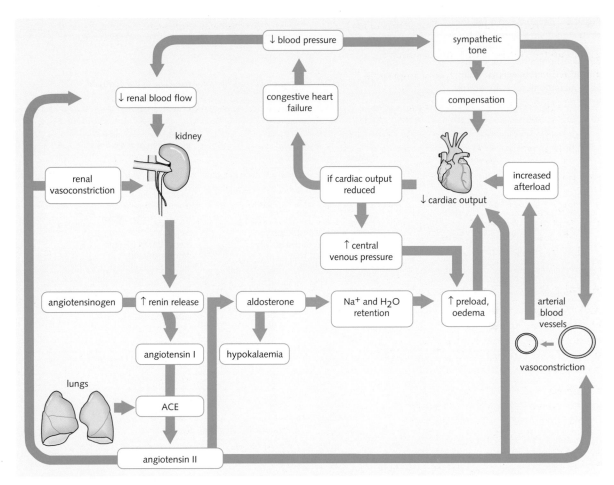

Fig. 4.7   Compensatory mechanisms in congestive cardiac failure. ACE, angiotensin-converting enzyme.

Cardiogenic shock

This occurs when the heart fails to maintain cardiac output acutely (e.g. ischaemic heart disease, arrhythmias). As a result, tissue perfusion decreases dramatically. Venous pressure increases, causing pulmonary or peripheral oedema (as described above). Prognosis is poor (90% mortality). Massive pulmonary embolisms and pericardial tamponade are also causes of shock.

Vasodilated shock

Sepsis, anaphylaxis and spinal trauma decrease the total systemic resistance and can reduce the blood pressure sufficiently to cause shock.

Hypovolaemic shock

This occurs when there is an acute reduction in effective circulating blood volume from blood loss (haemorrhage), loss of plasma (e.g. burns) or loss of water and electrolytes (e.g. diarrhoea and vomiting).

Figure 4.8 shows the response to a fall in circulating fluid volume. To counteract excessive vasoconstriction as a result of sympathetic activity in the kidneys, more vasodilating prostaglandins (PGE_2 and PGI_2) are secreted within the kidneys. This maintains adequate blood flow through the kidney to allow sufficient glomerular filtration, unless the shock is severe. The loss of large amounts of fluid has two major consequences:

- Volume depletion (decreases tissue perfusion)
- Electrolyte and acid–base disturbance.

As Na^+ is involved in the co-transport of H^+, K^+ and Cl^-, the acid–base balance is disturbed because Na^+ is retained. Cl^- is reabsorbed in equal quantities but, initially, there is increased secretion of H^+ and K^+, resulting in metabolic alkalosis (contraction alkalosis) and hypokalaemia. This is balanced by the shift to anaerobic metabolism as a result of hypoxia in the tissues, which eventually prevails to cause a metabolic acidosis. This is further potentiated as hypovolaemia becomes more severe, as less urine is excreted and H^+ is no longer excreted.

61

Fig. 4.8 Response to a fall in circulating fluid volume. ACE, angiotensin-converting enzyme; BP, blood pressure; CO, cardiac output; ECF, extracellular fluid; JGA, juxtaglomerular apparatus.

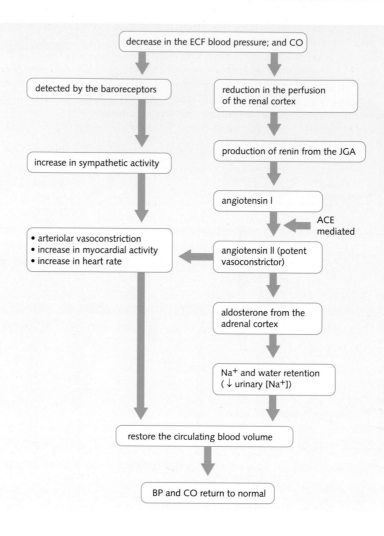

Treatment

The treatment of hypovolaemic shock requires fluid replacement to restore the extracellular volume. If blood flow to the kidneys is not restored, acute kidney injury results from tissue anoxia and necrosis.

Hepatorenal syndrome

Patients with liver disease can have a reduced urine flow (oliguria). This is especially so in patients with portal hypertension and ascites. Portal hypertension results from an increase in resistance to blood flow from the gut and spleen, resulting in venous congestion. Possibly due to the release of nitric oxide, there is peripheral vasodilatation. The resulting decrease in blood pressure causes sympathetic activation and activation of the renin–angiotensin–aldosterone system, leading to intense renal vessel vasoconstriction which leads to oliguira and renal failure.

The circulating blood volume can also be reduced in liver disease from the formation of ascites and oedema. These result from portal hypertension and the impaired synthesis of albumin, decreasing the oncotic (colloid osmotic) pressure in the capillaries, favouring fluid movement out of the vsculature. These shifts in fluid out of the vasculature can contribute to the acute kidney injury.

Hypertension

Blood pressure (BP) is influenced by the interaction of genetic and environmental factors, which regulate cardiac output (CO) and total peripheral resistance (TPR):

$$BP = CO \times TPR$$

The kidneys influence blood pressure by regulating the volume of extracellular fluid (ECF). They also release vasoactive substances:

- Vasoconstrictors: angiotensin II
- Vasodilators: prostaglandins.

Renal autoregulation maintains renal function despite variations in systolic blood pressure. Any change in the ECF will affect the blood pressure. The kidney compensates for these changes by controlling Na^+ and water excretion. If this mechanism is disturbed there will be uncontrolled Na^+ and water retention, resulting in hypertension. Hypertension is defined by the World Health Organization as a sustained blood pressure of 140/90 mmHg or above.

Essential hypertension

This accounts for about 95% of all cases of hypertension and the cause is unknown. Initially, there is an increase in cardiac output as a result of sympathetic overactivity. In the later stages the increase in blood pressure is maintained by an increase in the total peripheral resistance, but cardiac output is normal. Hypertensive changes seen in the kidney include:

*   Arteriosclerosis of the major renal arteries
*   Hyalinization of the small vessels with intimal thickening.

This can lead to chronic renal damage (hypertensive nephrosclerosis) and a reduction in the size of the kidneys.

Malignant or 'accelerated' hypertension is a rare and rapidly progressing form of severe hypertension. It is characterized by fibrinoid necrosis of the blood vessel walls, and ischaemic damage to the brain and kidney. This can lead to acute renal failure or heart failure, requiring urgent treatment.

Secondary hypertension

This is caused by renal (80%) and endocrine diseases, and occasionally drugs (ciclosporin).

Renal causes
Renal mechanisms causing hypertension include:

*   Impaired sodium and water excretion, increasing blood volume
*   Stimulation of renin release.

Most diseases of the kidney disease can result in hypertension, e.g. diabetic nephropathy, any cause of glomerulonephritis, chronic pyelonephritis and polycystic kidney disease. Renal artery stenosis (discussed below) causes reduced perfusion of the kidney and therefore excessive activation of the renin–angiotensin system.

Clinical Note

The kidneys influence blood pressure by regulating ECF volume, and also release vasoactive substances:
*   Vasoconstrictors: angiotensin II
*   Vasodilators: prostaglandins.

Endocrine causes
The endocrine causes are:

*   Cushing's syndrome
*   Oestrogen (i.e. the contraceptive pill and pregnancy)
*   Phaeochromocytoma (rare)
*   Primary hyperaldosteronism (Conn's syndrome).

In primary hyperaldosteronism there is chronic excessive secretion of aldosterone because of an adrenal cortical adenoma or hyperplasia (Fig. 4.9). Patients present with hypertension and hypokalaemia. Diagnosis is made based on the triad of:

*   Hypokalaemia
*   Increased aldosterone
*   Decreased renin.

Treatment is by surgical removal of the adenoma, with a cure rate of 60% on aldosterone antagonists (spironolactone). Recent studies have suggested that hyperaldosteronism may be a more common cause of hypertension than previously realized.

Drug causes
Corticosteroids, the combined oral contraceptive pill, NSAIDs and ciclosporin can all cause hypertension.

Coarctation of the aorta
A congenital narrowing of the aorta reduces renal perfusion and thus stimulates the renin–angiotensin–aldosterone system.

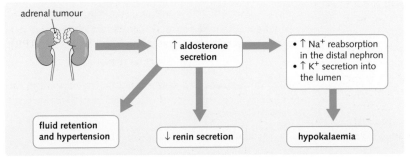

Fig. 4.9 Mechanism by which an adrenal tumour (Conn's syndrome) causes secondary hypertension.

Management of hypertension

It is difficult to detect and treat hypertension because it is often asymptomatic and many patients are reluctant to take medication if they feel well. It is very important to exclude an underlying cause of hypertension.

Hypertension is an important risk factor for strokes, cardiac failure, myocardial infarction and chronic kidney disease. Effective treatment will improve the prognosis for each of these conditions. NICE guidelines are available for the treatment of hypertension.

Lifestyle changes include:

- Weight reduction
- Reduced alcohol intake
- Salt restriction
- Regular exercise
- Smoking cessation.

Drug treatment of hypertension involves:

- Diuretics
- ACE inhibitors

- Ca^{2+} channel blockers
- β-blockers (now not first-line).

Angiotensin-converting enzyme inhibitors (ACE i)

These inhibit ACE, and so block formation of angiotensin II. Angiotensin II is a potent vasoconstrictor and promotes sodium reabsorption in the tubule (Fig. 4.10). ACE inhibitors (e.g. captopril, ramipril) lower blood pressure by:

- Reducing total peripheral resistance
- Inhibiting the local (tissue) renin–angiotensin system.

ACE inhibitors also reduce proteinuria and delay the progress of renal disease in patients with diabetic nephropathy and patients with proteinuric non-diabetic renal disease. They are also used to treat CCF.

The side-effects of ACE inhibitors include:

- Persistent dry cough
- Allergic reactions or rashes

Fig. 4.10 Effects of ACE (angiotensin-converting enzyme) inhibitors. +ve, positive feedback; −ve, negative feedback.

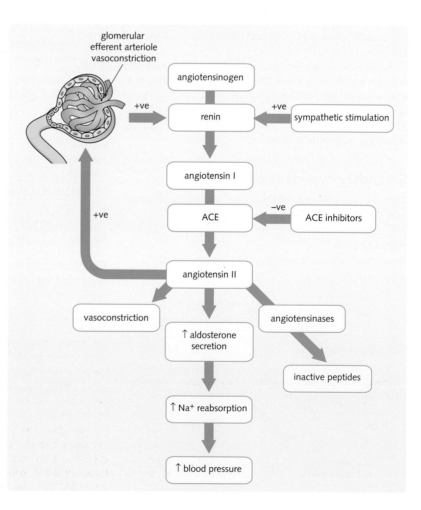

- Changes in the sensation of taste
- Severe hypotension especially in patients who are hypovolaemic
- Acute renal failure in patients with renal artery stenosis (renal function should be checked after giving ACE inhibitors)
- Hyperkalaemia.

ACE inhibitors are contraindicated in pregnancy because of the risk of:

- Developmental abnormalities in the fetal kidney
- Oligohydramnios (reduced amniotic fluid)
- Neonatal hypotension and anuria.

> **HINTS AND TIPS**
>
> ACE inhibitors prevent the breakdown of bradykinin by ACE. This is thought to be the cause of the dry cough they commonly cause. In this case angiotensin II receptor blockers (ARBs) can be used which do not cause the increase in bradykinins.

Diuretics

Diuretics increase the volume of urine produced by increasing renal sodium excretion (natriuresis), which is followed passively by water. Each type of diuretic has specific actions on the normal physiology of a particular segment (Fig. 4.11):

- Act on the membrane transport proteins found on the luminal surface
- Interfere with hormone receptors
- Inhibit enzyme activity.

Osmotic diuretics

Osmotic diuresis can be induced by an inert substance that is not reabsorbed in the tubule. The proximal tubule and the descending limb of the loop of Henle allow free movement of water molecules. If an agent such as mannitol is introduced into the tubular fluid, it is not absorbed and thus reduces water reabsorption. There is increased urine flow through the nephrons resulting in reduced sodium reabsorption. Osmotic diuretics are used to:

- Increase urine volume when renal haemodynamics are compromised, and thus prevent anuria
- Reduce intracranial pressures in neurological conditions
- Reduce intraocular pressures before ophthalmic surgery.

Excessive use of osmotic diuretics without adequate fluid replacement can cause dehydration and hypernatraemia.

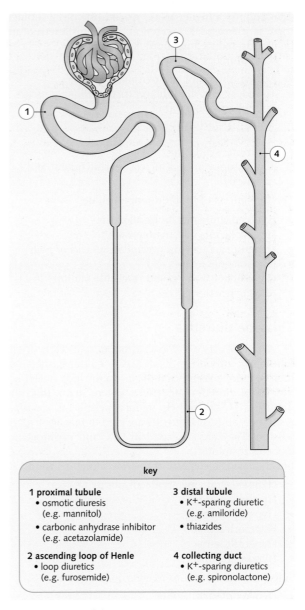

key	
1 proximal tubule • osmotic diuresis (e.g. mannitol) • carbonic anhydrase inhibitor (e.g. acetazolamide)	**3 distal tubule** • K$^+$-sparing diuretic (e.g. amiloride) • thiazides
2 ascending loop of Henle • loop diuretics (e.g. furosemide)	**4 collecting duct** • K$^+$-sparing diuretics (e.g. spironolactone)

Fig. 4.11 Sites of diuretic action.

Loop diuretics

These are the most powerful diuretics, causing up to 20% of filtered Na$^+$ to be excreted. They inhibit sodium transport out of the thick ascending limb of the loop of Henle into the medullary interstitium. Examples include furosemide and bumetanide. Loop diuretics act by inhibiting the Na$^+$/K$^+$/2Cl$^-$ co-transporter on the luminal membrane of the cells. This inhibits Na$^+$ reabsorption, thereby diluting the osmotic gradient in the medulla. This results in increased Na$^+$ and water excretion. Positive lumen potential falls as cations are retained, causing an increase in Ca^{2+} and Mg^{2+}

excretion. As a higher $[Na^+]$ reaches the distal tubule, there is increased K^+ secretion, so loop diuretics can be used to reduce total body K^+.

Loop diuretics are used for:

- Acute pulmonary and peripheral oedema
- To reduce end-diastolic ventricular filling pressure
- Pulmonary congestion
- Acute hypercalcaemia
- Hypertension
- Nephrotic syndrome
- Acute kidney injury (increases urine output and K^+ excretion).

The side-effects of loop diuretics include:

- Hypokalaemic metabolic alkalosis
- Hypovolaemia and hypotension
- Hyperuricaemia (can precipitate attacks of gout)
- Hypomagnesaemia
- Ototoxicity (dose-related reversible auditory loss)
- Allergic reactions.

Thiazide diuretics

These reduce active Na^+ reabsorption in the early distal tubule by inhibiting the Na^+/Cl^- co-transporter. As there is more reabsorption of Na^+ in the loop of Henle, the loop diuretics are more potent than thiazide diuretics. Thiazides help reduce peripheral vascular resistance, and consequently are used to manage hypertension. They are also used in CCF and nephrogenic diabetes insipidus.

Renal-related side-effects of thiazide diuretics include:

- Hypokalaemic metabolic alkalosis
- Hyperglycaemia
- Hyperlipidaemia
- Hyperuricaemia
- Hypercalcaemia
- Hyponatraemia.

Side-effects unrelated to renal actions include:

- Hypercholesterolaemia
- Reversible male impotence
- Allergic reactions (rare).

HINTS AND TIPS

Side effects of thiazide diuretics: Hyper GLUC (hyper glucose, lipid, uric acid and calcium).

Potassium-sparing diuretics

These diuretics are K^+-sparing and act:

- In the collecting ducts (e.g. spironolactone)
- By inhibiting the uptake of Na^+ in the cells of the distal nephron (e.g. amiloride and triamterene).

Aldosterone is a mineralocorticoid that increases the activity of the Na^+/K^+ ATPase, potassium and sodium channels, resulting in Na^+ absorption and K^+ secretion.

Spironolactone (a mineralocorticoid analogue) competes with aldosterone for the receptor site. This reduces sodium reabsorption in the distal nephron and decreases K^+ secretion (potassium-sparing activity).

Potassium-sparing diuretics are used if there is mineralocorticoid excess such as primary aldosteronism (Conn's syndrome) or ectopic ACTH production. They are also used in secondary aldosteronism where salt and water retention have occurred (e.g. CCF, nephrotic syndrome, liver disease and hypovolaemia). They are fairly weak, often used with loop diuretics or thiazides to prevent K^+ loss.

The side effects include:

- Hyperkalaemia: this results from an increase in H^+ – and therefore K^+ – retention as Na^+ absorption falls and ranges from mild to life-threatening
- Endocrine effects with spironolactone (e.g. gynaecomastia).

Potassium-sparing diuretics are contraindicated in patients with chronic renal insufficiency.

Carbonic anhydrase inhibitors

Carbonic anhydrase (CA) is found in many places in the nephron but primarily on the brush border of the luminal membrane of the proximal tubule cells. CA catalyses the dehydration of H_2CO_3:

$$H^+ + HCO_3^- \leftrightharpoons H_2CO_3 \leftrightharpoons H_2O + CO_2$$

This reaction is driven by H^+ secretion into the lumen, by cotransport with Na^+. Once in the cell, H_2CO_3 is reformed under the influence of intracellular CA, the HCO_3^- ions are reabsorbed, and H^+ is secreted back into the lumen (see Fig. 3.5).

CA inhibitors interfere with the action of carbonic anhydrase and inhibit HCO_3^- reabsorption. The presence of HCO_3^- in the lumen reduces Na^+ reabsorption, which continues into the distal nephron where it enhances K^+ secretion.

CA inhibitors such as acetazolamide are weak diuretics, which cause the excretion of only about 5–10% of the filtered Na^+ and water. Their main clinical use is to treat acute and chronic glaucoma by reducing intraocular pressure (the production of aqueous humour in the eye involves secretion of HCO_3^- by the ciliary body in a process similar to that in the proximal tubule).

The side-effects of CA inhibitors include:

- Metabolic acidosis
- Renal stones
- Renal K^+ wasting
- Nervous system effects – paraesthesia and drowsiness.

CA inhibitors should be avoided in patients with liver disease or late-stage CKD.

DISEASES OF THE RENAL BLOOD VESSELS

Renal artery stenosis

Between 2% and 5% of hypertensive patients have hypertension secondary to narrowing of one or both renal arteries. This reduces the pressure in the afferent arterioles, which stimulates the juxtaglomerular apparatus to secrete renin. The affected, ischaemic kidney is small. There are two types:

- Atherosclerotic renovascular disease: Atherosclerosis accounts for 70% of renal artery stenosis. It may be suspected when there is other evidence of vascular disease e.g. femoral or aortic bruits, coronary artery disease, peripheral vascular disease, aortic aneurysms. It may be asymptomatic
- Fibromuscular dysplasia: This is usually seen in young women and can often be cured with renal artery angioplasty and stenting (Fig. 4.12).

It may present with hypertension, suddenly decreasing renal function with ACE inhibitors, a renal bruit or recurrent flash pulmonary oedema from fluid retention. Treatment options include:

- Drugs to control the blood pressure and vascular risk factors: If the blood pressure is left uncontrolled the contralateral kidney may become damaged by hypertension. ACE inhibitors can be used cautiously to reduce the effect of the renin–angiotensin–aldosterone system, but renal function must be monitored carefully. It is essential to control vascular risk factors and aspirin and a statin should be considered and smoking cessation advised
- Angioplasty: to dilate the stenotic region. This can be supplemented with stenting to decrease the risk of restenosis. This is most successful for fibromuscular dysplasia but the benefit in atherosclerotic renal artery disease is less clear.

Fig. 4.12 Comparison between fibromuscular dysplaisa and atheromatous renal artery stenosis (RAS).

	Fibromuscular dysplasia	Atheromatous RAS
Age (years)	<40	>55
Sex prevalence	F > M	M > F
Bruit heard	80%	40%
Vascular disease	Rare	Common elsewhere
Renal failure	Rare	Well recognized
Prognosis	Good	Poor

Clinical Note

ACE inhibitors and ARBs can cause a significant reduction of renal function in patients with renal artery stenosis. Carefully monitored, however, they are the ideal antihypertensive therapies to prevent further glomerular damage.

Thrombotic microangiopathies

This is a group of diseases that are all characterized by necrosis and thickening of the renal vessel walls and thrombosis in the interlobular arterioles, afferent arterioles and glomeruli. All clinically present with the triad of:

- Haemolysis
- Thrombocytopenia
- Acute kidney injury.

The main two microangiopathies are:

1. Haemolytic uraemic syndrome (HUS)
2. Thrombotic thrombocytopenic purpura (TTP).

Haemolytic uraemic syndrome

This is characterized by the triad of:

- Microangiopathic haemolytic anaemia
- Thrombocytopenia (decreased platelets)
- Acute kidney injury (with normal clotting).

It is classified as:

- **Idiopathic**: this is more common in adults, and has a worse prognosis
- **Secondary**: this can be associated with gastroenteritis (e.g. *Escherichia coli* 0157 toxin), drugs (oestrogen, ciclosporin, cytotoxic therapy) or malignancy. HUS can also be caused by accelerated hypertension. There may also be a genetic cause.

Clinical features include sudden onset of oliguria with haematuria – occasionally with melaena or haematemesis (usually if gastroenteritis is the cause) – and jaundice. Hypertension is seen in 50% of patients.

Treatment involves early supportive therapy with dialysis for renal failure. Fresh frozen plasma or plasma exchange can be useful. Approximately 50% of patients later develop hypertension, and a few go on to develop CKD. Mortality ranges from 5% to 30%.

Thrombotic thrombocytopenic purpura

This is a rare and idiopathic condition that is more common in females (usually < 40 years) than in males. The features are fever, neurological signs (central nervous system (CNS) involvement), haemolytic anaemia and thrombocytopenia. TTP has a similar disease process to HUS, but affects different sites. Renal involvement occurs in only 50% of cases, and presents with:

- Proteinuria
- Haematuria
- Renal insufficiency.

The majority of cases have a dominant CNS component, with thrombosis leading to ischaemia in the brain.

Histological examination shows thrombi consisting of fibrin and platelets in the terminal interlobular arteries, the afferent arterioles and glomerular capillaries.

Treatment involves corticosteroid therapy and plasma exchange.

Renal infarction

Embolic infarction

The embolus can come from:

- Thrombotic material from the left side of the heart
- Atheromatous material from plaques
- Bacterial vegetations from infective endocarditis.

The emboli lodge in the small renal vessels and cause narrowing of the arterioles and focal areas of ischaemic injury. It can be asymptomatic, or present with haematuria and loin tenderness. The areas of infarction appear pale and are characteristically wedge-shaped.

Diffuse cortical necrosis

Diffuse cortical necrosis is caused by profound hypotension. Typical causes are sepsis or hypovolaemia following severe blood loss. It presents with anuria and carries a very poor renal prognosis.

Sickle-cell disease nephropathy

Thrombotic occlusion by deformed sickle-shaped red cells causes papillary necrosis. It is precipitated by cold, dehydration, infection and exercise. Presentation is with pain, haematuria and polyuria. Management involves analgesia, warmth and rehydration, blood transfusions and antibiotics (if infection is suspected).

Benign nephrosclerosis

This is the term given to the changes in renal vasculature in response to longstanding essential (benign) hypertension. The changes consist of hyaline arteriolosclerosis, which is characterized by thickening (due to hyperplasia of smooth muscle) and hyalinization (protein deposition) of the arteriolar wall. This causes narrowing of the lumen of the interlobular arteries, which functionally impairs the smaller branches. The changes are more severe in patients with systemic diseases that affect the renal vessels (e.g. diabetes). The vascular wall lesions gradually reduce the blood supply to the kidney, which leads to ischaemic atrophy of the nephrons. This accounts for the small, contracted and granular appearance of the kidneys seen in advanced cases of untreated essential hypertension. Renal function may be well-preserved initially, although proteinuria is sometimes detected.

Malignant nephrosclerosis

This is associated with accelerated hypertension, with an increase in diastolic pressure to over 130 mmHg. There are fibrin deposits in the vessel wall, causing necrosis, especially in the distal part of the interlobular arteries and the afferent arterioles.

Renal function is impaired because of the ischaemia that results from severe arterial damage. Patients have proteinuria and haematuria, which can occasionally be massive. Acute kidney injury develops if untreated (in contrast to benign hypertension). Papilloedema is often present. The 5-year survival rate with treatment is more than 50%.

The trigger for the abrupt and rapid rise in blood pressure is unknown but might be associated with endothelial dysfunction. These patients also have increased plasma levels of renin, aldosterone and angiotensin.

Clinical Note

Benign hypertension causes glomerular damage and small contracted kidneys.

Malignant hypertension leads to acute kidney injury through malignant nephrosclerosis.

The lower urinary tract 5

Objectives

By the end of the chapter you should be able to:
- State two qualities of urothelium that make it suitable to line the bladder and ureters
- Outline the function of the detrusor and sphincter muscles, and their innervations
- Describe the embryological origin and significance of double and bifid ureters
- Summarize common neurological causes of difficulties with micturition
- Explain the difference between stress and urge incontinence
- List the causes of urinary obstruction and explain the significance of hydronephrosis
- List the five types of urinary calculus and their causes
- State the maximum diameter of calculus generally considered likely to pass spontaneously
- Give the risk factors and symptoms of acute cystitis and list the common UTI pathogens
- Outline the mechanism by which schistosomiasis increases the risk of bladder cancer
- Understand the causes of inflammation of the prostate
- Define benign prostatic hyperplasia and explain the histological changes

ORGANIZATION OF THE LOWER URINARY TRACT

Overview

Urine formed in the kidneys collects in the renal pelvis and then passes down the lower urinary tract (ureters, bladder and urethra) before exiting the body. The bladder stores the urine, which is ejected intermittently from the body under voluntary control.

Ureters

The ureters are hollow muscular tubes 25–30 cm long, which begin as funnel-shaped tubes at the renal pelvis. They run retroperitoneally over the posterior abdominal wall in front of the external iliac artery down to the pelvic brim (similar course in the female). Figs 5.1 and 5.2 show the course of the ureters through the pelvis in a man and woman, respectively. As urine collects in the renal pelvis, the pelvis dilates. Action potentials in the pacemaker cells of the renal pelvis are set up, stimulating peristaltic contractions in the ureters that propel the urine.

The ureters are divided into regions related to their anatomical course: renal pelvis, abdominal, pelvic and intramural regions (Fig. 5.3). This influences the source of blood supply to each region of the ureter – renal, lumbar segmental, gonadal, common iliac, internal iliac and superior vesical arteries, with corresponding venous drainage.

The ureters are innervated by both sympathetic and parasympathetic nerves. As shown in Figure 5.3 there are constrictions in the ureters. Stones can get stuck at these constrictions and produce acute colicky pain, which is referred to the skin of T11–L2. Therefore, pain starts in the loin and radiates to the scrotum and penis (men) or to the labium majora (women).

Histologically, the ureter has three layers of smooth muscle (see Fig. 5.3):
- A longitudinal layer just outside the lumen
- A middle circular layer
- Another longitudinal layer.

The lumen is lined by urothelium (also known as transitional epithelium), which is folded in the relaxed state, allowing the ureter to dilate during the passage of urine. The plasma membranes of urothelium are thicker than other cell membranes, preventing interstitial fluid from entering the concentrated urine. Urothelium is impermeable to urine. The cells have highly interdigitating cell junctions, allowing the epithelium to stretch without damaging the surfaces of the cells. It also lines the bladder and prostatic urethra.

HINTS AND TIPS

Reflux of urine from the bladder back into the ureter is prevented by a valvular mechanism at the vesicoureteric junction. If the valve is incompetent, urinary reflux occurs and chronic pyelonephritis can ensue.

Fig. 5.1 Anatomy of the male lower urinary tract.

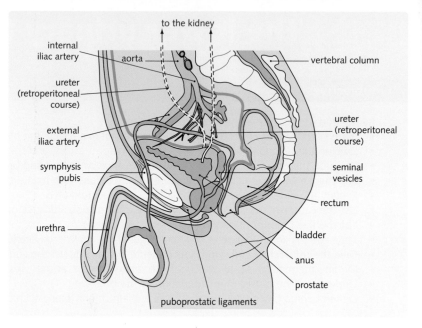

Fig. 5.2 Anatomy of the female lower urinary tract.

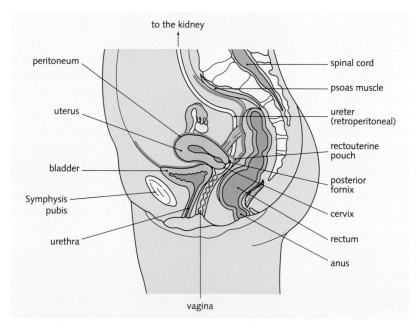

Urinary bladder

The ureters enter the base of the bladder, which is partially covered by peritoneum.

- When empty it lies in the pelvis and rests on the symphysis pubis and floor of the pelvis
- When filled, it enlarges into the abdominal cavity.

The neck of the bladder is relatively immobile and fixed by the puboprostatic and lateral vesical ligament. The blood supply to the bladder is from the superior and inferior vesical branches of the internal iliac artery. It is drained by the vesical plexus and by the prostatic venous plexus in the male, which then drain into the internal iliac vein. Lymphatic drainage is also along

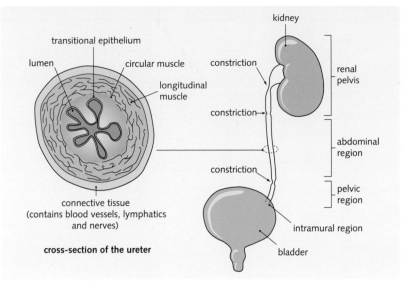

Fig. 5.3 Regions of the ureter and cross-sectional view. The normal points of reduced diameter are also shown, at which stones commonly lodge.

the vesical blood vessels to the internal iliac nodes, then the para-aortic nodes.

Interior of the bladder

The wall is yellow with rugae (folds), lined by transitional epithelium, allowing expansion with little increase in internal pressure. The base is the trigone, which is a triangular, reddish region bounded by the ureteric openings into the bladder and the internal urethral meatus (see Fig. 5.4). This area is less mobile and less distensible than the rest of the bladder. It is more sensitive to painful stimuli.

The bladder is lined by smooth muscle, known as the detrusor muscle, which, like the ureter, is arranged in spiral, long and circular bundles. Smooth muscle bundles surround the bladder neck to form the internal urethral sphincter. Slightly further along the urethra there is a skeletal muscle sphincter – the external urethral sphincter.

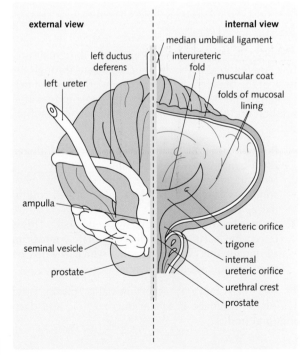

Fig. 5.4 Posterior and interior view of the male bladder.

> ### HINTS AND TIPS
>
> • The internal urethral sphincter is not under voluntary control and thus contracts reflexively
> • The external urethral sphincter is under voluntary control.

Bladder innervation (Fig. 5.5) is both:

• **Sensory**: gives sensation (awareness) of a full bladder and also pain from disease. The impulses are suppressed if the bladder is empty

• **Motor**: parasympathetic activity stimulates the detrusor muscle, so the bladder contracts. It also inhibits the external urethral sphincter, which relaxes to allow micturition. Sympathetic activity inhibits the detrusor muscle, so the bladder relaxes, and stimulates the urethral sphincter (this contracts). Both these actions prevent micturition.

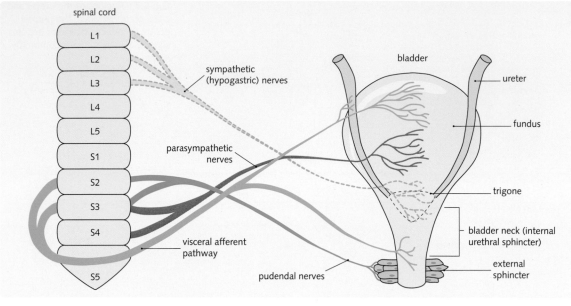

Fig. 5.5   Innervation of the bladder. (From Koeppen BM, Stanton B, 1996. Renal physiology, 2nd edn. Mosby Year Book.)

Male urethra

The male urethra (Fig. 5.6) is longer than the female urethra (male = 20 cm, female = 4 cm). It runs through the neck of the bladder, the prostate gland, the floor of pelvis and the perineal membrane to the penis and external urethral orifice at the tip of the glans penis. It has three parts:

1. Prostatic urethra: surrounded by prostate tissue, lined by transitional epithelium
2. Membranous urethra: the shortest region, with sphincter activity, lined by pseudostratified columnar epithelium
3. Spongy urethra: surrounded by penile tissue. This is lined by pseudostratified columnar epithelium except for the external opening which is lined by stratified squamous epithelium.

It is innervated by the prostatic plexus and lymphatic drainage is to the internal iliac and deep inguinal nodes.

Female urethra

This starts at the neck of the bladder and passes through the floor of the pelvis and perineal membrane to open into the vestibule just anterior to the opening of the vagina. It is 4 cm in length and is firmly attached to the anterior wall of the vagina. Lymphatics drain to the internal and external iliac lymph nodes. Proximally it is lined by transitional epithelium and the rest by stratified squamous epithelium.

Prostate

This is a gland lying below the bladder in the male and surrounding the proximal part of the urethra (prostatic urethra). It measures $4 \times 3 \times 2$ cm and is conical in shape. It is connected to the bladder by connective tissue stroma and has three parts:

1. Left lateral lobe
2. Right lateral lobe
3. Middle lobe.

The prostate has a connective tissue capsule, which is surrounded by a thick sheath from the pelvic fascia. It is influenced by sex hormones resulting in growth during puberty. As the prostate surrounds the urethra, any enlargement can narrow the urethra and obstruct urine flow.

The prostate is supplied by the inferior vesical artery and blood drains via the prostatic plexus to the vesical plexus and internal iliac vein. Lymphatics drain to the internal iliac and sacral nodes.

The prostate contains a central zone of mucosal glands originating prenatally from the endoderm. These drain directly into the urethra. There is also a peripheral zone of mucosal glands, derived from the mesoderm, which drains into the ducts that enter the urethral sinus. Prostatic glandular epithelium can vary from inactive low cuboidal cells to active pseudostratified columnar cells, depending on the degree of androgen stimulation from the testes. The glands secrete 75% of seminal fluid, which is thin, milky and rich in citric acid and hydrolytic enzymes (e.g. fibrinolysin). This prostatic secretion liquefies coagulated semen after deposition in the

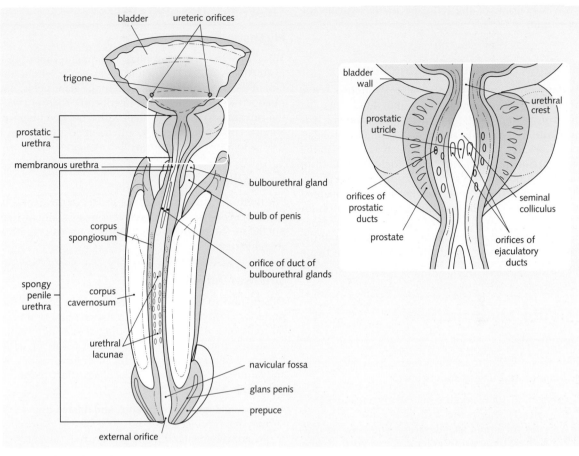

Fig. 5.6 The male urethra.

female genital tract. The prostate is covered by a stroma and capsule made of dense fibroelastic connective tissue with a smooth muscle component.

Renal function is rarely affected but there is a strong predisposition to infection. Urine can reflux from the bladder, especially through the upper pole ureter. Treatment

CONGENITAL ABNORMALITIES OF THE URINARY TRACT

Ureteric abnormalities

Double and bifid ureters

The ureters along with the calyces and collecting ducts are formed from an outgrowth of the mesonephric (Wolffian) duct called the ureteric bud. Early splitting of the ureteric bud or the development of two buds results in duplication, which can be:

- Partial: the two ureters meet before entering the bladder together. These are called bifid ureters
- Complete: the two ureters enter the bladder separately. The upper pole ureter enters the bladder lower and more medially than the lower ureter. These are called double ureters (see Fig. 5.7).

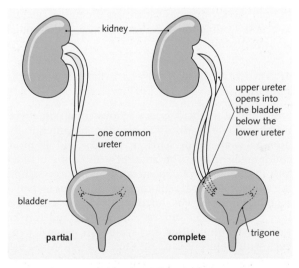

Fig. 5.7 Partial and complete bifid ureter.

involves excision of the refluxing ureter (usually the upper one).

Pelviureteric junction obstruction

This often presents in infancy, although milder forms might not present until later in adult life or may be found in asymptomatic patients at postmortem. It is more common in males and in the left ureter. It is bilateral in 20% of cases, and might present as a mass in the flank or pain after drinking. It is thought to result from abnormal smooth muscle organization at where the renal pelvis joins the upper ureter. It can be accompanied by renal agenesis of the opposite kidney; the reason for this is unknown. As a result of the back pressure from the obstruction, the pelvicalyceal system dilates. If the pressure is transmitted to the kidneys, the renal tissue atrophies.

Bladder abnormalities

Diverticula

These are sac-like outpouchings through a weak point in the bladder wall. They can be either:

- Congenital: these develop in localized areas of defective muscle within the wall or because of urinary tract obstruction in fetal development. They are usually solitary lesions, most commonly occurring close to the ureterovesical junction
- Acquired: these usually develop much later in life as a result of chronic urethral obstruction (e.g. prostatic hypertrophy). They are clinically significant and, characteristically, occur as multiple lesions.

In both cases, urine stasis increases the risk of bladder infection, leading to vesicoureteric reflux and eventual stone formation.

Exstrophy

Exstrophy of the bladder is a serious condition affecting the anterior wall of the bladder and anterior abdominal wall. It presents in infancy and is more common in males. The anterior wall of the bladder fails to develop, so the posterior wall lies exposed on the lower abdominal wall, causing squamous metaplasia of the mucosa. The mucosa is at high risk of infection. This disorder can vary in severity and can be associated with urethral and symphysis pubis defects. Even with surgical treatment there is an increased risk of adenocarcinoma of the bladder later in life, because of bladder extrusion.

Urethral abnormalities

Hypospadias

This is a spectrum of congenital abnormalities affecting 1 in 400 male infants. The urethra opens on the ventral surface of the penis, usually adjacent to the glans penis, but can open on the penile shaft or perineum. There is a ventral curvature to the penile shaft with a hooded prepuce. Surgical correction is usually carried out before the age of 2 years to allow micturition with a straight stream.

Epispadias

The urethra opens on the dorsal surface of the penis. As with hypospadias, surgical correction is usually carried out before the age of 2 years to allow micturition with a straight stream.

Urethral valves

Obstruction to urine flow can occur at the level of the posterior urethra in a boy due to the presence of mucosal folds or a membrane extending across the urethra (posterior urethral valve). The patient presents in early infancy with distended bladder, dribbling, vomiting and failure to thrive. As a result of obstruction to urinary flow, male fetuses can have:

- Poor renal growth with reflux and dilated upper urinary tracts
- Progressive bilateral hydronephrosis
- Oligohydramnios (reduced volume of amniotic fluid).

Intrauterine intervention has no proven benefit and an early delivery is performed only if there are signs of rapidly progressing renal damage. Postnatal management includes:

- Prophylactic antibiotics from birth to prevent urinary tract infections (UTI)
- Ultrasound scans at birth and a few weeks later to assess the effect of the obstruction.

Surgical treatment is required in all cases.

> **HINTS AND TIPS**
>
> Any male child born with bilateral hydronephrosis must be investigated for a posterior urethral valve.

MICTURITION

Normal micturition

Micturition is the intermittent voiding of urine stored in the bladder. It is an autonomic reflex that is under voluntary control. The inside of the bladder wall is folded

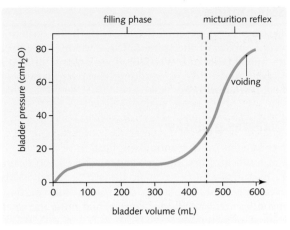

Fig. 5.8 Normal cystometrogram showing the rise in pressure associated with increasing bladder volume.

and can expand and accommodate fluid with little increase in pressure. However, it can accommodate only a certain volume of fluid before an increase in intravesical pressure occurs, causing an urge to micturate. Fig. 5.8 shows a normal cystometrogram in which pressure rise is compared with rise in volume in the bladder.

Fig. 5.5 shows the innervation of the bladder. In infants, micturition is a local spinal reflex in which the bladder empties on reaching a critical pressure. However, in adults this reflex is under voluntary control, so can be inhibited or initiated by higher centres in the brain. During micturition:

- Perineal muscles and the external urethral sphincter relax
- The detrusor muscle contracts (parasympathetic activity)
- Urine flows out of the bladder.

Bladder distension with urine stimulates bladder stretch receptors, which, in turn, stimulate the afferent limb of voiding reflex and parasympathetic fibres of the bladder, resulting in the desire to urinate. Higher-centre stimulation of the pudendal nerves keeps the external sphincter closed until it is appropriate to urinate. Fig. 5.9 illustrates the voluntary control of micturition.

Neurological disorders of micturition

Urinary continence is affected by various neurological lesions along the micturition pathway as summarized in Fig. 5.10.

Lesion in the superior frontal gyrus

This can be the result of a stroke and leads to:

- Reduced desire to urinate
- Difficulty stopping micturition once started.

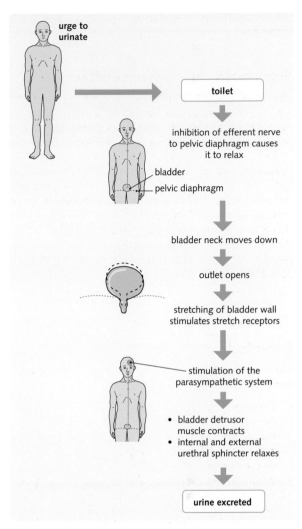

Fig. 5.9 Voluntary control of micturition.

Lesion of afferent nerves from the bladder

A lesion of afferent nerves from the bladder (e.g. caused by disease of the dorsal roots such as tabes dorsalis) prevents reflex contractions of the bladder, so the bladder becomes distended, thin-walled and hypotonic.

Lesion of both afferent and efferent nerves

A lesion of both afferent and efferent nerves (e.g. because of a tumour of the cauda equina or filum terminale) results in:

- Initially: bladder flaccidity and distension
- Later: bladder hyperactivity with dribbling.

This leads to a shrunken bladder with a hypertrophied bladder wall.

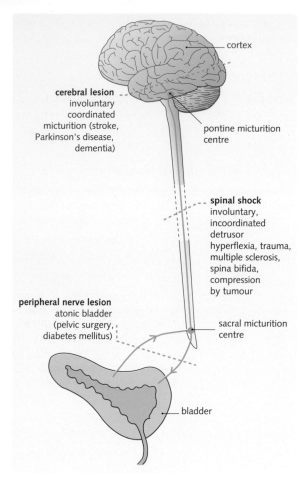

Fig. 5.10   Sites of damage along the micturition pathway.

Spinal cord lesion

A lesion to the spinal cord above the sacral micturition centre (e.g. spinal shock sustained following trauma) results in:

- Initially: overflow incontinence, because of a flaccid and unresponsive bladder, which results in overfill and dribbling. This is spinal shock
- After shock has passed: the voiding reflex returns, but with no control from higher centres, so the patient has no voluntary control over voiding
- Occasionally: hyperactive voiding might be seen
- Eventually: bladder capacity falls and the wall hypertrophies – spastic neurogenic bladder.

HINTS AND TIPS

Spinal cord injuries lead to reflex micturition, as is seen in infants. This occurs because patients with spinal cord lesions cannot synchronize detrusor muscle contractions with sphincter relaxation.

Spina bifida

This is a developmental defect in which the posterior neural arches of the spine fail to develop, so part of the spinal cord and its coverings are exposed. It forms a spectrum of defects, resulting in varying degrees of bladder dysfunction.

Diabetes mellitus

Neuropathy is a common complication of diabetes. It can result in a loss of sensation, so there is no desire to micturate and the patient voids infrequently. This eventually leads to bladder distension, with overflow incontinence. The presence of residual urine increases the risk of infection.

Multiple sclerosis

This is demyelination of white matter. The bladder symptoms that develop depend on the level at which demyelination occurs.

Pelvic surgery

The nerve supply to the bladder can be injured during surgery, resulting in postoperative urinary retention. This is usually transient.

Urinary incontinence

Urinary incontinence is the involuntary loss of urine. It affects more women than men and is a socially distressing condition. There are several different types.

Stress incontinence

This is involuntary leakage of small amounts of urine associated with an increase in intra-abdominal pressure (e.g. coughing, laughing, exercising). The sphincter is incapable of preventing the leakage. It is caused by:

- Pelvic floor laxity (usually the result of childbirth)
- Bladder neck sphincter impairment (more common in middle-aged, obese, multiparous women)
- Surgery affecting the urethra or prostate (e.g. TURP) causing damage or weakness to the external sphincter.

Pelvic floor exercise (e.g. Kegel) are an effective, non-invasive treatment but require cooperation and commitment from patients. Duloxetine, a serotonin and noradrenaline (norepinephrine) reuptake inhibitor, can be used for stress incontinence. There are a variety of options for surgical management, including tension-free vaginal tape (TVT) and transobturator tape (TOT) where the proximal urethra is lifted with an artificial sling, so that increases in intra-abdominal pressure compress the urethra.

Urge incontinence

This is the sudden strong urge to void followed immediately by involuntary loss of urine. It is part of overactive bladder syndrome, caused by detrusor overactivity. Causes include:

- Damage to the nervous system innervating the detrusor muscle, such as stroke, Parkinson's disease, Alzheimer's disease
- Inflammation of the lower urinary tract from infection or stones.

The management of detrusor instability involves the behavioural techniques of bladder drill and training, regulating then increasing the amount of time between voiding. Antimuscarinic medication, e.g. Oxybutynin is also used.

> **HINTS AND TIPS**
>
> The detrusor muscle is the bladder muscle and contracts to cause voiding. This is an automatic reflex, triggered by filling of the bladder to a critical pressure.

Overflow incontinence

This is involuntary leakage of urine when the bladder is full. It is usually due to chronic urinary retention secondary to obstruction or an atonic bladder. The causes are:

- Outlet obstruction: faecal impaction, benign prostatic hypertrophy (enlarged prostate)
- Underactive detrusor muscle
- Bladder neck stricture
- Urethral stricture
- α-Adrenergic agonists
- Use of anticholinergics, calcium channel blockers, sedatives
- Bladder denervation following surgery.

Continuous incontinence

This is the continuous loss of urine at all times. The causes are:

- Vesicovaginal fistulae, secondary to gynaecological surgery, obstetric injury, radiation or tumours
- Ectopic ureter, bypassing urine from the kidneys to the urethra or vagina, uncontrolled by any sphincter.

Functional incontinence

This is incontinence due to severe cognitive impairment or mobility limitations, preventing use of the toilet. For example, there might be difficulty in reaching the toilet or difficulty in undressing, and the patient is 'caught short'. Bladder function is normal.

Mixed incontinence

In mixed incontinence there is more than one type of problem resulting in incontinence. This is usually seen in older patients.

Nocturnal enuresis – bedwetting

Nocturnal enuresis is a childhood disorder. It can be primary (since birth) or secondary. Both can be due to:

- Uninhibited bladder activity
- Urinary infection
- Neurological disease
- Obstruction.

After urinary tract infection has been excluded, no further investigation should be performed if the child is under 5 years – unless there are any urinary symptoms. Treatment should focus on behaviour therapy with star charts or alarms that wake the child when starting to micturate. Drug treatment with desmopressin, an ADH analogue, is a last resort.

URINARY TRACT OBSTRUCTION AND UROLITHIASIS

Urinary tract obstruction

Obstruction in the urinary tract can occur at any level. It can be unilateral or bilateral, complete or incomplete, and of gradual or acute onset. It increases the risk of UTI, reflux and stone formation. If prolonged or unrelieved, obstruction can cause functional renal impairment and permanent renal atrophy.

Fig. 5.11 shows the sites of obstruction in the urinary tract. Obstruction is caused by a congenital defect or, more commonly, by a structural lesion.

Congenital abnormalities

These include the following neuromuscular defects:

- Urethral valves and strictures
- Meatal strictures
- Bladder neck obstruction
- Ureteropelvic obstruction or stenosis.

Mechanical obstruction of the meatus and urethra occurs only in boys. Severe vesicoureteric reflux eventually results in upper renal tract dilatation without obstruction.

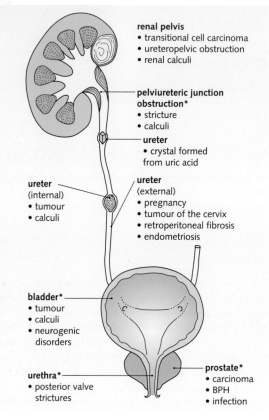

renal pelvis
• transitional cell carcinoma
• ureteropelvic obstruction
• renal calculi

pelviureteric junction
obstruction*
• stricture
• calculi

ureter
• crystal formed
from uric acid

ureter
(internal)
• tumour
• calculi

ureter
(external)
• pregnancy
• tumour of the cervix
• retroperitoneal fibrosis
• endometriosis

bladder*
• tumour
• calculi
• neurogenic
disorders

urethra*
• posterior valve
strictures

prostate*
• carcinoma
• BPH
• infection

Fig. 5.11 Sites of obstruction in the urinary tract.* The most common sites of obstruction. BPH, benign prostatic hyperplasia.

Tumours

Tumours can cause obstruction in two ways:

1. Internal: tumours within the urinary tract wall or lumen (e.g. bladder carcinoma). These occupy the urinary tract lumen, causing direct obstruction
2. External: pressure from rectal or prostate tumours or from gynaecological malignancies narrows the urinary tract lumen, causing indirect obstruction.

Calculi (urolithiasis)

Stones in the urinary tract can cause urinary obstruction.

Pregnancy

The high levels of progesterone in pregnancy relax smooth muscle fibres in the renal pelvis and ureters and cause a dysfunctional obstruction. There might also be external compression from the pressure of the enlarging fetus on the ureters.

Hyperplastic lesions

The most common hyperplastic lesion causing urinary obstruction is benign prostatic hypertrophy (BPH).

Inflammation

Any inflammation in the lower urinary tract will cause an obstruction (e.g. urethritis, ureteritis, prostatitis, retroperitoneal fibrosis). Obstruction resolves with the treatment of the inflammation.

Neurogenic disorders

These result from:

• Congenital anomalies affecting the spinal cord (e.g. spina bifida)
• External pressure on the cord or lumbar nerve roots (e.g. meningioma, lumbar disc prolapse)
• Trauma to the spinal cord.

Hydronephrosis

This is dilatation of the renal pelvis and calyces due to obstruction at any point in the urinary tract causing increased pressure above the blockage. It can be:

• Unilateral: caused by an upper urinary tract obstruction. This is detected late because renal function is maintained by the other kidney. Thus, the affected kidney can be severely impaired by the time obstruction is detected
• Bilateral: because of obstruction in the lower urinary tract. Renal failure develops earlier and prompt intervention is required to prevent chronic kidney disease.

Progressive atrophy of the kidney develops as the back pressure from the obstruction is transmitted to the distal parts of the nephron. The glomerular filtration rate (GFR) declines and, if the obstruction is bilateral, the patient goes into renal failure. Progressive damage to the renal structures results in flattening of the calyces with gradual thinning of the renal parenchyma, eventually leaving a cystic, thin-walled, fibrous sac with no functional capacity.

Clinical Note

• Obstruction at the pelviureteral junction: hydronephrosis
• Obstruction of the ureter: hydroureter, eventually developing hydronephrosis
• Obstruction of the bladder neck/urethra: bladder distension with hypertrophy, eventually leading to hydroureter and thus hydronephrosis. If bilateral, renal failure develops earlier.

Presentation of urinary obstruction

This depends on the site and cause of the obstruction:

- An acute complete obstruction in the ureters (e.g. due to a stone) causes severe pain (renal colic). Only if bilateral, will the patient develop acute renal impairment
- Gradual obstruction (e.g. prostatic hypertrophy) causes bladder distension with hesitancy, terminal dribbling, poor urine flow and a sense of incomplete voiding
- A unilateral and partial obstruction causing a hydro-ureter or hydronephrosis might not be apparent for many years because the unaffected kidney maintains adequate renal function
- A bilateral and partial obstruction presents with nocturia and polyuria caused by tubular cell dysfunction with an inability to concentrate urine. Other chronic manifestations include renal stones, salt wasting, distal renal tubular acidosis and hypertension. If undiagnosed, the patient develops chronic renal failure
- A bilateral and complete obstruction presents as anuria or oliguria and must be treated urgently. Following removal of the obstruction, there may be a post-obstructive diuresis which can result in dehydration if not managed appropriately. Any general malaise or fever might be a sign of superimposed infection.

In all cases, the prompt and effective relief of the obstruction is essential to preserve the renal parenchyma. Depending on the site this may require a urinary catheter, urinary stent or a nephrostomy (to allow renal function to improve), followed by surgical intervention.

> **HINTS AND TIPS**
>
> - Sudden and complete obstruction causes a fall in GFR, resulting in acute kidney injury
> - Partial or chronic obstruction does not affect the GFR, so renal function is impaired gradually.

Urolithiasis (urinary calculi)

Urinary calculi affect 10% of the population and are more common in men and Caucasians. Stone formation is initiated by a core of mucoproteins or urates (nucleation); as more components precipitate on the core, the stone gradually increases in size (aggregation). Dehydration increases the concentration of the urine hence is a predisposing factor.

There are five main types of calculi:

- Calcium oxalate stones, the most common cause (Fig. 5.12). These are associated with hypercalcaemia

Fig. 5.12 Different types of calculus and their frequency.

Type	Frequency (%)
Calcium-containing stones:	
Calcium oxalate	75
Mixed calcium phosphate and calcium oxalate	10
Magnesium ammonium phosphate	15
Uric acid stones	5
Cystine stones	1–2

and primary hyperparathyroidism and hyperoxaluria. The absence of citrate in the urine predisposes to these stones
- Mixed calcium phosphate and calcium oxalate stones. These are associated with alkaline urine, caused by renal tubular acidosis types 1 and 3
- Magnesium ammonium phosphate stones (MAP, struvite, infection stones), associated with urea-splitting bacteria, e.g. *Proteus mirabilis*
- Uric acid stones, associated with gout and myeloproliferative disorders
- Cystine stones occur in patients who have inherited (autosomal recessive) cystinuria.

They can form anywhere in the urinary tract. Occasionally, a calculus can grow to take up the shape of the renal pelvis and branch into calyces (staghorn calculus). The three most common sites for ureteric stones are:

- Pelviureteric junction
- Pelvic brim
- Vesicoureteric junction.

Presentation

The clinical presentation depends on the site of the stone:

- Renal stones may cause a continuous dull ache in the loins
- Ureteric stones cause classic renal colic due to the increase in peristalsis in the ureters in response to the passage of a small stone. This pain typically radiates from the loin to groin. The patient appears sweaty, pale and restless, with nausea and vomiting
- Bladder stones cause strangury: the urge to pass something that will not pass
- Recurrent and untreatable UTIs, haematuria or renal failure
- They may be asymptomatic.

CT scan of the kidneys, ureters and bladder is now the gold standard for diagnosing stones (all but uric acid stones are radio-opaque). Intravenous urogram does still have advantages, as it is less expensive and gives a lower radiation dose (see Chapter 8).

Treatment

Management involves adequate analgesia and a high fluid intake. The urine should be sieved for analysis. Stones of 5 mm or less in diameter usually pass spontaneously; larger stones might require surgical intervention. Tamsulosin and nifedipine increase the likelihood of stones passing. Other treatment options include:

- Extracorporeal lithotripsy: shock waves are used to fragment the calculi into small pieces which will then pass out in the urine
- Ureteroscopic destruction or removal of stones
- Percutaneous surgery: endoscopic removal of the stone
- Open surgical removal.

Prevention of further stone formation is achieved with a high fluid intake and correction of any underlying metabolic abnormality.

Clinical Note

Urgent treatment of stones is needed if there is decreasing renal function, infection with urinary obstruction or bilateral obstruction.

INFLAMMATION OF THE URINARY TRACT

Cystitis

Inflammation of the bladder (cystitis), as part of urinary tract infection (UTI) is very common. If it involves loin pain and fever this indicates infection of the kidneys (pyelonephritis), discussed in Chapter 3. UTIs are more common in boys in infancy because of congenital abnormalities; this reverses at puberty, with more females being affected thereafter because of urethral trauma and pregnancy. Women are particularly at risk of cystitis because they have a short urethra, but further investigation is required if infections are recurrent. Any UTI in children and men should be investigated to exclude an underlying renal tract abnormality. UTIs rarely progress to renal damage in adults if the renal tract is normal. After the age of 40, UTI again becomes more common in men because of prostatic disease, causing bladder outflow obstruction. Risk factors for cystitis include:

- Urethral catheterization
- Diabetes mellitus

Fig. 5.13 Incidence of community-and hospital-acquired urinary tract infections (UTIs) caused by bacteria.

Organism	Community (%)	Hospital (%)
Escherichia coli	80–90	45–55
Proteus	5–10	10–12
Klebsiella	1–2	15–20
Enterobacter	–	2–5
Pseudomonas	–	10–15
Acinetobacter	–	<1
Coagulase-negative Staphylococcus	1–2	1–2
Staphylococcus aureus	–	<1
Enterococcus	<1	10–12

- Impaired voiding (due to obstruction)
- Pregnancy
- Sexual intercourse
- Tumours
- Immunosuppression.

The typical irritative symptoms of cystitis are dysuria (pain on passing urine), frequency and urgency of micturition and suprapubic pain.

A diagnosis of UTI requires over 10^5 organisms/mL from a midstream urine specimen. In the majority of UTIs the infecting organism comes from the patient's own faecal flora (Fig. 5.13). Treatment involves a high fluid intake, regular bladder emptying and antibiotics.

Non-infective cystitis can be caused by radiation, drugs (e.g. cyclophosphamide, ketamine) and instrumentation.

Chronic cystitis

This results from recurrent or persistent infection of the bladder. Chronic infection leads to fibrous thickening, so the bladder wall is less distensible. This affects the ability of the bladder to store urine and contract during micturition.

Interstitial cystitis

This type of cystitis is often associated with systemic lupus erythematosus, so is thought to be an autoimmune condition. As with all autoimmune conditions, it has a much higher incidence in women than in men. It can also result from recurrent and persistent infection that leads to fibrosis of all the layers of the bladder wall. There is often localized ulceration of the mucosa.

Malakoplakia vesicae

This is a very rare form of chronic bacterial cystitis, but it is important because it can mimic a tumour. Raised mucosal plaques of inflammation cells develop on the bladder and ureteric mucosa. These plaques are soft, yellow, 3–5 cm in diameter and are prone to ulceration.

Schistosomiasis (bilharzia)

Schistosomiasis is the most common helminth infection worldwide, although it is rare in the UK. It is endemic in the Middle East, Africa, the Far East and in parts of South America. The pathogen is a blood fluke (*Schistosoma haematobium*). Freshwater snails are also part of its complicated life cycle. The schistosomes penetrate intact skin to enter the venous system, and migrate to the liver and bladder. They settle in the bladder to lay eggs causing chronic irritation of the transitional cells of the bladder. The eggs are excreted into local water supplies and transmitted through freshwater snails (Fig. 5.14).

People infected with cercariae can present with an itchy papular rash accompanied by myalgia, abdominal pain and headache. The most common presentation of infection with *S. haematobium* is recurrent haematuria. Eventually, urinary tract obstruction, bladder calcification (predisposing to squamous carcinoma) and CKD can occur.

Diagnosis involves:

- Urine sample to detect the eggs in the urine
- Enzyme-linked immunosorbent assay (ELISA) on serum to detect an antibody response to infection.

Treatment is with praziquantel given once daily.

> **Clinical Note**
>
> Squamous metaplasia associated with chronic bladder inflammation and schistosomiasis is a premalignant condition, leading to squamous cell carcinoma.

Urethritis

Acute inflammation of the urethra occurs from infection with a sexually transmitted disease (e.g. *Neisseria gonorrhoeae* or *Chlamydia trachomatis*) (see *Crash Course: Endocrine and Reproductive System* for further details). It can be related to urethral diverticuli, urethral carbuncles or phimosis and can result in urethral stricture.

DISORDERS OF THE PROSTATE

Prostatitis

There are three subgroups of inflammation of the prostate.

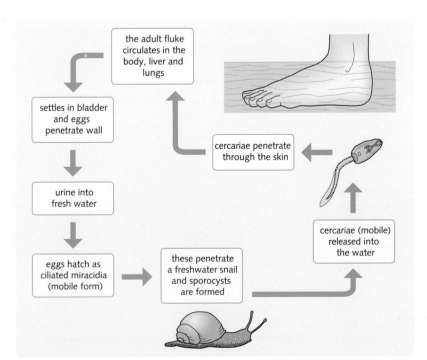

Fig. 5.14 Infestation with *S. haematobium*.

Acute prostatitis

The main pathogens are *E. coli*, *Proteus* and *Staphylococcus* species, and sexually transmitted pathogens including *C. trachomatis* and *Neisseria gonorrhoeae*. Inflammation can be focal or diffuse. Infection is usually spread from an acute infection in the urethra or bladder because of:

- Intraprostatic reflux of urine
- Intraprostatic catheterization
- Surgical manipulation of the urethra (e.g. cystoscopy).

Occasionally, acute prostatitis is caused by a blood-borne infection.

On histological examination there is an acute inflammatory infiltrate of neutrophils and damaged cells, often resulting in abscess formation.

Patients present with:

- General symptoms: malaise, rigours and fever
- Local symptoms: difficulty in passing urine, dysuria and perineal tenderness.

Rectal examination reveals a soft, tender and enlarged prostate. Diagnosis is based on the clinical features and a positive urine culture.

Chronic prostatitis

This results from inadequately treated acute infection. This can occur because some antibiotics cannot penetrate the prostate effectively. There is often a history of recurrent prostatic and urinary tract infections. Causative pathogens are the same as for acute prostatic infection.

Patients present with dysuria and low back and perineal pain, with no preceding acute phase. Some patients are asymptomatic.

Chronic prostatitis is difficult to diagnose and treat. Diagnosis is confirmed by:

- Histological examination showing neutrophils, plasma cells and lymphocytes
- A positive culture from a sample of prostatic secretion.

Tuberculosis is a cause of chronic infection and can affect the kidneys or epididymis. Histological examination reveals focal areas of caseation and giant cell infiltrates.

Chronic non-bacterial prostatitis

This is the most common type of prostatitis and results in enlargement of the prostate, which can obstruct the urethra. The usual pathogen is *C. trachomatis* so, typically, sexually active men are affected. Often there is no history of recurrent UTIs.

Presentation is similar to that of chronic prostatitis and histological examination shows fibrosis as a result of chronic inflammation.

Diagnosis is confirmed by the presence of 15 white blood cells per high-power field (this indicates inflammation) and repeated negative bacterial cultures (excludes infection).

Benign prostatic hypertrophy

Incidence

BPH is detectable to some extent in nearly all men over the age of 60. It is a non-neoplastic enlargement of the prostate gland, which can eventually lead to bladder outflow obstruction. The cause is unknown, but might be related to levels of male sex hormones (testosterone).

Presentation

Symptoms develop as the enlarging gland compresses the prostatic urethra and the periurethral glands (known as the median lobe) swell, affecting the bladder sphincter mechanism. Men present with obstructive lower urinary tract symptoms (LUTS):

- Difficulty or hesitancy in starting to urinate
- A poor stream
- Dribbling postmicturition
- Frequency and nocturia.

These symptoms can be caused by other conditions, shown in Fig. 5.15. Examination must include:

- Abdominal examination for an enlarged palpable bladder
- Digital rectal examination for the prostate, which is firm, smooth and rubbery.

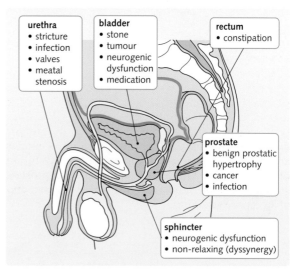

Fig. 5.15 The causes of obstructive lower urinary tract symptoms.

Untreated BPH can present with acute urinary retention, which is accompanied by a distended and tender bladder and a desperate urge to pass urine. Alternatively, the patient might have progressive bladder distension, leading to chronic painless retention and overflow incontinence. If undetected, BPH can lead to bilateral upper tract obstruction and renal impairment, with the patient presenting in chronic kidney disease (see Chapter 7).

Clinical Note
Enlarging of the prostate gland in BPH presents with:
- Hesitancy in starting urination
- Poor stream
- Dribbling postmicturition
- Frequency
- Nocturia.

Pathology

There is hyperplasia of both the lateral lobes and the median lobes (these lie behind the urethra), leading to compression of the urethra and therefore bladder outflow obstruction. Within the prostate there are solid nodules of fibromuscular material and cystic regions. Histological examination shows hyperplasia of the:

- Stroma (smooth muscle and fibrous tissue)
- Glands, often with areas of infarction and necrosis.

Complications

The complications of BPH develop from prolonged obstruction to urine flow. There is compensatory hypertrophy of the bladder as a result of the high pressures that develop within the bladder (Fig. 5.16).

Treatment

Medical treatment
Symptoms can be improved with α-blockers which relax smooth muscle at the bladder neck and within the prostate, thus improving urinary flow rate. Finasteride is a 5a-reductase inhibitor that prevents the conversion of testosterone to the more potent androgen dihydrotestosterone. Dihydrotestosterone promotes growth and enlargement of the prostate so inhibition of its production causes gradual reduction in prostate volume, thereby improving urinary flow rate and obstructive symptoms.

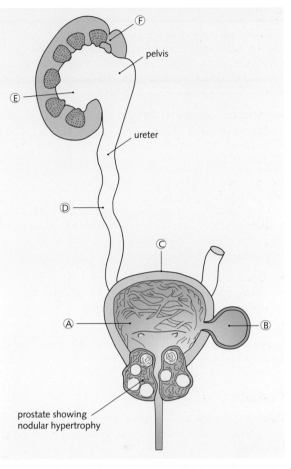

Fig. 5.16 Complications of benign prostatic hypertrophy. (A) Bands of thickened smooth muscle fibres cause trabeculation of the bladder wall. (B) Diverticula can develop on the external surface of the bladder. (C) Dilatation of the bladder once the muscle becomes hypotonic. (D) Formation of hydroureters resulting in the reflux of urine up to the renal pelvis. (E) Bilateral hydronephrosis. (F) Kidney infection, stones, calculi and renal failure.

Surgical treatment
Transurethral resection of the prostate (TURP) is the most common operation for BPH. Complications include haematuria, retrograde ejaculation and impotence. A dilutional hyponatraemia can be seen following TURP as a result of absorbance of water and glycine from irrigation fluid used during the procedure. This can lead to a 'transurethral resection syndrome' of confusion, vomiting, hypertension and visual disturbance.

Neoplasia and cysts of the urinary system

Objectives

By the end of the chapter you should be able to:
- Outline the epidemiology of renal cell carcinoma
- Discuss the paraneoplastic conditions related to renal cell carcinoma
- Describe Wilms' tumour
- Outline the mechanism by which schistosomiasis increases the risk of bladder cancer
- Recognize the common presentation of bladder cancer
- Explain how treatment and prognosis differ according to the stage of prostate cancer
- Understand the genetics of adult polycystic kidney disease
- Discuss how the prognosis in adult polycystic kidney disease differs from that in childhood polycystic kidney disease

NEOPLASTIC DISEASE OF THE KIDNEY

Benign tumours of the kidney

These rarely cause symptoms and are usually found as an incidental finding on CT, ultrasound or post mortem.

Renal fibroma or hamartoma

This is the most common benign renal tumour. It is a small (less than 1 cm diameter) firm, well-demarcated, white nodule in the medulla. The nodule is composed of spindle cells and collagen. It is often an incidental finding with no clinical significance.

Cortical adenoma

This is a small (<1 cm diameter) discrete, yellowish-grey tumour derived from renal tubular epithelium. It is an incidental finding in 20–25% of post mortems. On histological examination it is found to be composed of large vacuolated clear cells with small nuclei (this is also seen in renal cell carcinoma).

HINTS AND TIPS

It is often difficult to differentiate benign cortical adenomas from malignant renal cell carcinomas, radiologically and pathologically. Even masses smaller than 3 cm have malignant potential.

Malignant tumours of the kidney

Renal cell carcinoma

Incidence and risk factors

Approximately 90% of renal malignant tumours in adults are renal cell carcinomas (RCCs); they arise from the tubular epithelium. RCCs are rare in children and have a peak incidence in 60–70-year-olds. The male to female ratio is 3:1. There is great geographical variance with the highest incidence in Scandinavia and the lowest in South America and Africa. Risk factors are:

- Acquired cystic disease in patients who require renal replacement therapy – RCC tends to occur at a much earlier age in these patients
- Von Hippel-Lindau disease: this is a rare autosomal dominant condition caused by a mutation on chromosome 25; 50–70% of these patients develop RCC
- Smoking.

Presentation

Approximately 90% of cases present with haematuria. Non-specific symptoms include fatigue, weight loss and fever. There might be a mass in the loin. These are all late manifestations, presenting at an advanced stage of tumour progression, at which time prognosis is poor. RCCs often metastasize before local symptoms develop.

A small number of RCCs can secrete hormone-like substances such as:

- Parathyroid hormone, resulting in hypercalcaemia
- Adrenocorticotrophic hormone (ACTH), resulting in a Cushing's-like syndrome
- Erythropoietin, resulting in polycythaemia
- Renin, resulting in hypertension.

As a result of producing hormones, RCC can present with paraneoplastic syndromes.

Diagnosis
Diagnosis is by:

- IVU: this reveals a space-occupying lesion in the kidney that distorts the outline
- Ultrasonography: this distinguishes between solid and cystic lesions
- CT: provides preoperative staging (see Chapter 8).

Pathology
RCC consists of a yellow-brown, well-demarcated mass in the renal cortex, with a diameter of 3–15 cm. Within this area there are patches of haemorrhage, necrosis and cyst formation. The tumours are most common at the upper pole of the kidney. The renal capsule is often intact, although it can be breached and the tumour will extend into the perinephric fat. Spread into the renal vein is often visible and rarely this extends into the inferior vena cava.

Histological examination reveals cells with clear cytoplasm that range from well differentiated to anaplastic.

Spread occurs by direct invasion of local tissues, via the lymph to lumbar nodes (a third of cases), and via the blood (venous). Metastases are found in the lung, liver, bone, opposite kidney and adrenals.

Prognosis
Prognosis depends on tumour size and the degree of the spread; RCC staging involves assessing local, nodal and metastatic spread (TNM classification).

T_1: <7 cm and confined to the kidney
T_2: >7 cm with distortion of the kidney with renal capsule intact
T_3: spread through the renal capsule into the perinephric fat with invasion into the renal vein
T_4: invasion into adjacent organs or the abdominal wall
N^+: lymph node involvement
M^+: metastatic spread.

Treatment
For large tumours with no distant metastases treatment involves a radical nephrectomy with removal of the associated adrenal gland, perinephric fat, upper ureter and the para-aortic lymph nodes. Postoperative radiotherapy is required to decrease risk of recurrence. Increasingly, small tumours are removed with a partial nephrectomy to preserve some renal function on that side. There is little effective treatment available for metastatic disease. The average 5-year survival rate is 45%, increasing up to 70% if there is no metastatic disease at diagnosis.

Wilms' tumour (nephroblastoma)
Incidence and presentation
This is the most common malignant renal tumour in children. The peak incidence is in 1–4-year-olds, with both sexes affected equally. It is an embryonic tumour derived from the primitive metanephros. It presents with an abdominal mass and occasionally haematuria, abdominal pain and hypertension.

Pathology
The tumours are large solid masses of firm white tissue with areas of necrosis and haemorrhage. They often breach the renal capsule and grow into the perinephric fat. Histological examination reveals spindle cells or primitive blastema cells with epithelial and mesenchymal tissues, cartilage, bone and muscle. They are aggressive tumours, often presenting with metastatic disease of the lung.

Treatment and prognosis
Treatment involves nephrectomy, radiotherapy and chemotherapy. The long-term survival rate is over 80%.

Prognosis depends upon tumour size and distant spread at the time of diagnosis.

Urothelial carcinoma of the renal pelvis
This is a transitional cell tumour accounting for 5–10% of renal tumours. It can be caused by:

- Analgesic misuse
- Exposure to aniline dyes used in the industrial manufacture of dyes, rubber and plastics.

Presentation with haematuria or obstruction occurs early, because the renal pelvis projects directly into the pelvicalyceal cavity. Fragments of papillary tumour and atypical tumour cells can be detected in the urine and this makes cytological diagnosis possible.

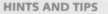

HINTS AND TIPS

Metastases from lymphomas, lung or breast cancer or melanomas can deposit in the kidneys.

NEOPLASTIC DISEASE OF THE URETERS AND BLADDER

Tumours of the ureters

These are rare.

Benign tumours of the ureter

These originate from blood vessels, lymphatics and smooth muscle. A fibroepithelial polyp is a small mass that projects into the lumen. It consists of a clump of vascular connective tissue beneath the ureteric mucosa.

Malignant tumours of the ureters

Primary malignancies are rare and metastatic disease is relatively more common in the ureters. Malignant tumours arise from the transitional epithelium lining the ureters and most of the urinary tract. They are usually asymptomatic for many years and are found in 60–70-year-olds. They eventually present as a partial and unilateral obstruction as the ureteric lumen becomes occluded. They often occur in association with multiple tumours of the bladder and renal pelvis (synchronous tumours of the urothelium).

Tumours of the bladder

Metaplasia

The transitional cell lining (urothelium) of the bladder can undergo metaplastic changes during any period of infection or inflammation as a result of stones, drugs and radiation. There are three types of metaplasia:

1. Squamous metaplasia: this occurs in areas of long-term chronic inflammation in bladder exstrophy, bladder calculi, and schistosomiasis. It is a risk factor for squamous cell carcinoma
2. Intestinal or glandular metaplasia: this is associated with chronic cystitis and leads to the formation of slit-like glands of columnar epithelium
3. Nephrogenic metaplasia (rare): this is associated with chronic infections. The urothelium is transformed to cuboidal epithelium, and must be differentiated from adenocarcinoma.

Benign tumours of the bladder

These are very rare. Transitional cell papillomas can be inverted or exophytic. Inverted papillomas consist of solitary nodules in the mucosa and measure 1–3 cm in diameter. Exophytic papillomas are small projections (0.5–2.0 cm in length) with uniform cellular structure. Papillary tumours are more likely to be grade I transitional cell carcinomas.

Transitional cell carcinoma of the bladder

These are malignant tumours that arise from the transitional cell epithelium that lines the bladder. They account for over 90% of bladder epithelial cell tumours,

and the number of cases is increasing. They are uncommon under 50 years of age and more commonly affect males (4 males : 1 female).

> **Clinical Note**
>
> The most common urinary tract malignancy is transitional cell carcinoma and the most common site is the bladder. In countries where schistosomiasis is endemic, squamous cell carcinoma of the bladder is common.

Presentation

The most common presentation of any tumour of the bladder is painless haematuria. This is often accompanied by symptoms of a UTI (i.e. dysuria, frequency and urgency). Symptoms can also be caused by local invasion of the tumour causing ureteric obstruction. Risk factors include:

- Smoking
- Exposure to chemicals in the rubber industry (e.g. naphthylamine and benzidine)
- Analgesic misuse.

Pathology

There are two main types of transitional cell tumour (Fig. 6.1):

1. Papillary tumour (70%): this is a wart-like lesion covered in a thick layer of urothelium branching off a stalk that attaches it to the mucosa (as described above)
2. Sessile (flat) tumour: these are plaques of thickened mucosa with a well-defined border.

Both these types of tumour can be in situ or invasive:

- Carcinoma in situ (CIS): these are flat lesions that are confined to the mucosa of the upper urinary tract or bladder. They are the precursors of the invasive tumours

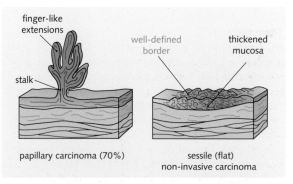

Fig. 6.1 Papillary and sessile transitional cell tumours.

- Invasive tumours: these infiltrate the basement membrane of the bladder mucosa and the lamina propria and can penetrate adjacent structures once through the mucosal wall.

Transitional cell carcinomas can be graded according to the degree of cellular abnormalities on histological examination:

- Grade I: there is an increase in the number of well-differentiated epithelial cell layers (>7) and there is some cell atypia
- Grade II: there is an increase in cell layers (>10) and there is a large variation in cell size and in nucleus shape and size (i.e. moderately well differentiated)
- Grade III: the cells have no resemblance to their cells of origin (poorly differentiated), with breakdown of connections between the cells causing them to fragment.

As tumour growth progresses, the relatively benign, well-differentiated papillary growths (grade I) can eventually form solid, plaque-like anaplastic tumours (grade III). Grade III tumours are often ulcerated and have penetrated through the bladder muscle wall. They are associated with the worst prognosis. Carcinomas with over 5% squamous or glandular metaplasia are called mixed tumours.

The TNM system is used for the staging of transitional cell tumours, i.e. to assess the extent of spread (Fig. 6.2). This has been correlated to grade. Tumour spread can be:

- Local: invasion into the bladder wall and to adjacent pelvic structures
- Distant: lymphatic spread to the periaortic lymph nodes or haematological metastases to the liver and lungs.

Investigation via cystoscopy and biopsy allows histological examination, which confirms whether there is muscle involvement. The distinction between the lamina propria invasion and submucosal invasion is correlated with the prognosis.

Most of the tumours are situated on the posterior and lateral walls of the bladder, and are often multiple. This suggests that the entire epithelium is unstable as a result of the constant exposure to the carcinogens being excreted in urine.

Diagnosis, treatment and prognosis

Diagnosis is made by cytological examination of the urine to check for the presence of malignant cells and by cystoscopy of the lower urinary tract.

Treatment depends on the stage and histological grade of the tumour:

- pTa/pT1 tumours: tumour resection using diathermy (via cystoscopy) with close follow-up
- pT2/3 tumours: radiotherapy and cystectomy
- pT4 tumours: palliative radiotherapy.

Intravesicular chemotherapy and intravesicular BCG (bacille Calmette Guérin) treatment have been shown to be effective in treating bladder cancer.

The average 5-year survival rate is 80% if the bladder wall is not involved and 5% if there is local invasion on presentation. Patients with fixed tumours and metastases have a median survival of 1 year.

Squamous cell carcinoma

These usually arise in areas of squamous metaplasia of the bladder mucosa and account for < 10% of bladder carcinomas. Risk factors include bladder exstrophy, chronic inflammation, calculi and schistosomiasis, which cause chronic irritation to the transitional cells of the bladder, leading to squamous metaplasia. This becomes dysplastic, resulting in carcinoma in situ, which can progress to invasive squamous cell carcinoma.

The tumours are solid, ulcerative, invasive and fungating masses, and are often very extensive on discovery. Their prognosis is worse than that of transitional cell carcinoma.

Adenocarcinoma

This is rare in the bladder and usually occurs in the urachal remnants, at the apex of the bladder. Histological examination shows metaplasia of the transitional epithelium or cystitis cystica.

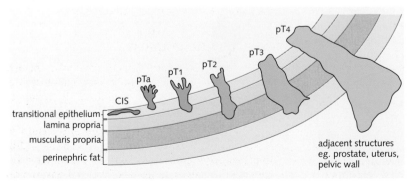

Fig. 6.2 TNM staging system for transitional cell carcinoma of bladder. T staging describes tumour invasion of the tissue layers; pT relating to the pathological staging proven by biopsy. N staging describes the degree of spread to the lymph nodes: N1, single node <2 cm; N2, single or multiple nodes <5 cm; N3, >5 cm. M staging describes the presence or absence of metastases: M0, none; M1, present. CIS, carcinoma in situ.

CARCINOMA OF THE PROSTATE

Incidence and risk factors

Prostate cancer is the most common cancer in men, accounting for 12% of all cancers. It is a disease of elderly men, occurring in 1 in 10 men of 70 years of age. It is rare under 55 years of age and has a strong hereditary component.

The lesions are most commonly found in the periphery of the posterior part of the prostate compared with the more central location of BPH (Fig. 6.3) – these areas have different embryological origins and often both conditions coexist.

Presentation

Patients present with symptoms of UTI, prostatism or metastatic disease in the bone (usually the spine) causing bone pain. Carcinoma can be found coincidentally in post mortems of elderly men who were asymptomatic. About 25% of patients have symptoms of metastatic disease on presentation (anaemia, ureteric obstruction or bone pain that is worse at night). Increasingly carcinoma

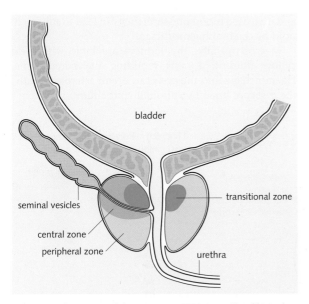

Fig. 6.3 The zones of the prostate. BPH typically affects the transitional zone so quickly causes obstruction of the urethra. Most prostatic carcinoma originates in the peripheral zone.

of the prostate is discovered following investigation of elevated prostate-specific antigen (PSA) in otherwise asymptomatic men. The value of early diagnosis in long-term outcome is currently unclear.

Pathology

The tumours range from well-differentiated single nodules to anaplastic and diffuse involvement of all lobes of the gland. The Gleason classification is used to grade the tumours on histological appearance. Grade 1 is a well-differentiated tumour composed of uniform tumour cells whereas grade 5 is an anaplastic diffuse tumour with cells showing great variation in their structure and a high mitotic rate.

Stage is determined by the TNM system:

- T_1: unsuspected impalpable tumour
- T_2: the tumour is confined to the prostate
- T_3: there is local extension of the tumour beyond the prostatic capsule
- T_4: the tumour has fixed to other local structures.

Tumour spread can be by:

- Local invasion of adjacent structures, including the bladder and ureters
- Lymphatic spread to the iliac and periaortic nodes
- Haematogenous spread to the bones of the spine and pelvis and occasionally to the lungs and liver.

Diagnosis

- Digital rectal examination: hard and irregular prostate
- Ultrasound: used to define a prostatic mass
- PSA level in the blood: this increases in prostate cancer, but a normal result does not exclude the presence of cancer
- Serum prostatic acid phosphatase: this also increases, especially if there are metastases
- Biopsy of the prostate (using a transrectal approach under ultrasound guidance (TRUS)) is required to provide a histological diagnosis
- Radiographs and bone scans: used to stage the tumour. Osteosclerotic lesions on radiographs and increased isotope uptake on bone scans are seen if there is metastatic spread (see Chapter 8).

Treatment and prognosis

Treatment options include surgery, hormone therapy and radiotherapy. Before treatment is started, a histological diagnosis of prostatic carcinoma is required. Treatment depends on the stage of the tumour:

- T1/T2 staged tumours: radical surgical resection of the prostate (prostatectomy) may be curative. TURP might also be required in advanced metastatic disease to relieve the symptoms of urethral obstruction

- Local radiotherapy can be used if the patient is unfit for surgery, and to treat local or distant spread of the tumour. It can provide useful palliation for bony metastases
- Advanced tumours: hormonal manipulation is beneficial since testosterone promotes tumour growth. Thus, removal of both testes (orchidectomy) blocking the source of testosterone, will cause the tumour to shrink, although this is rarely used now. Gonadotrophin-releasing-hormone (GnRH) analogues (e.g. goserelin) prevent testosterone release and are equally effective and are increasingly used. Antiandrogens such as cyproterone acetate are also used to block testosterone action.

Prognosis depends on stage. The 5-year survival rate for T1 tumours is 75–90%. However, the 5-year survival falls to 30–45% if there is local or metastatic spread.

CYSTIC DISEASES OF THE KIDNEY

Overview

Cystic diseases of the kidney include a spectrum of diseases comprising hereditary, developmental and acquired disorders. They can result if the ureteric bud or kidney tissue fails to develop. Some of these diseases can lead to chronic kidney disease (CKD). Diagnosis is made by finding multiple cysts on ultrasound. A single simple cyst is not an uncommon finding and should be considered normal.

Polycystic kidney disease

Adult – autosomal dominant

Incidence and presenting features
This type of polycystic kidney disease accounts for 8–10% of chronic kidney disease. Inheritance is autosomal dominant, and this is the most common inherited

nephropathy Three polycystic kidney disease (PKD) genes have been identified:

- *PKD 1:* on chromosome 16 (accounts for 85% of cases)
- *PKD 2:* on chromosome 4 (accounts for 10% of cases)
- *PKD 3:* accounts for a minority of cases and has yet to be mapped.

These mutations are thought to alter tubular epithelium growth and differentiation. Presentation is at 30–40 years of age with complications of hypertension, acute loin pain and/or haematuria, or bilateral large palpable kidneys. End-stage renal failure can develop, usually in the fifth or sixth decades of life. The disease is diagnosed increasingly earlier in life, as relatives of affected individuals are screened with abdominal ultrasound.

Pathology
Cysts develop anywhere in the kidney when dilatations in the nephron (Fig. 6.4A) compress the surrounding parenchyma and impair renal function. Sites for cyst formation are:

- Both kidneys
- Liver (lined by biliary epithelium) in 30–40% of cases
- Pancreas, lungs, ovaries, spleen and other organs.

Complications include uraemia, hypertension and berry aneurysms (found in 10–20% of cases). These develop as a result of congenital weakness in the arteries and increased blood pressure; they can lead to subarachnoid or cerebral haemorrhage.

Macroscopically, the kidneys are large with clear yellow fluid-filled cysts replacing the parenchyma. Haemorrhage into the cysts can occur. Microscopically, the cysts are lined by cuboidal epithelium.

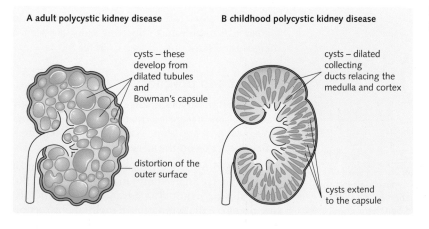

A adult polycystic kidney disease

cysts – these develop from dilated tubules and Bowman's capsule

distortion of the outer surface

B childhood polycystic kidney disease

cysts – dilated collecting ducts relacing the medulla and cortex

cysts extend to the capsule

Fig. 6.4 Polycystic (A) adult and (B) childhood kidney disease.

Diagnosis

Large, irregular kidneys, and possibly hepatomegaly, are found on physical examination. Diagnosis is made by ultrasound or computed tomography (CT): this shows bilateral enlarged kidneys with multiple cysts.

Prognosis

Morbidity and mortality are often the result of hypertension, for example myocardial infarction and cerebrovascular disease. The condition also leads to progressive chronic kidney disease (CKD). Rarely, complications are produced by the extrarenal cysts.

Treatment

This involves controlling blood pressure. Dialysis and renal transplant are needed if end-stage renal failure develops.

Child – autosomal recessive

Incidence and presenting features

This rare condition presents with enlarged kidneys or stillbirth. Both sexes are affected equally and more than one gene might be involved.

Pathology

Macroscopically, large kidneys with a radial pattern of fusiform-like cysts (sunburst pattern) are seen. Both kidneys are enlarged by multiple dilated collecting ducts which form the cysts. These replace the medulla and cortex and extend into the capsule (see Fig. 6.4B). The liver is almost always affected, with cysts, bile duct cell proliferation, fibrosis interfering with liver function and eventual portal hypertension.

Diagnosis, prognosis and treatment

Diagnosis is based on the presence of a palpable mass and ultrasound findings. Treatment involves managing the renal failure, hypertension and respiratory problems.

The prognosis is poor and death usually occurs due to renal or respiratory failure within the first few weeks of life, unless renal replacement therapy is given. Some children can survive for several years with independent renal function and develop portal hypertension and hepatic fibrosis.

Cystic renal dysplasia

This is an area of undifferentiated mesenchyme or cartilage within the parenchyma. It can be unilateral (better prognosis) or bilateral, and is often associated with obstructive abnormalities in the ureter and lower urinary tract. Presentation is in childhood as an abdominal mass, and it is treated with surgical excision.

Medullary sponge kidney

Incidence and presenting features

This is uncommon (1 in 20 000). It usually presents at 30–40 years of age with symptoms of urinary tract infection (UTI), stone formation or haematuria.

Pathology

Dilated collecting ducts in the medulla result in multiple cyst formation, mainly in the papillae (Fig. 6.5). Small calculi can develop within the cysts. One, part of one, or both kidneys can be affected. Macroscopically, some cysts are seen extending into the medulla from the involved calyces. In severe cases, the medulla looks spongy.

Fig. 6.5 *Medullary sponge kidney.*

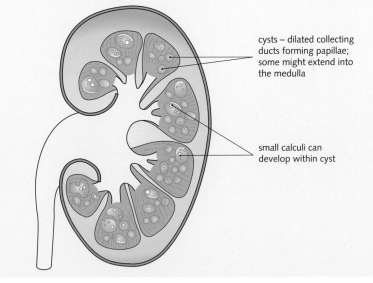

cysts – dilated collecting ducts forming papillae; some might extend into the medulla

small calculi can develop within cyst

Diagnosis, prognosis and treatment

Diagnosis is by intravenous urography (IVU) with cysts showing up as clusters of light. The prognosis is good, with renal function remaining intact. Treatment is treating and preventing infection and stone formation. A partial nephrectomy might be required.

Acquired cystic disease (dialysis associated)

Acquired cystic disease occurs in patients with CKD who have received dialysis for some time. The damaged kidneys develop many small cysts throughout the cortex and medulla, caused by obstruction of the tubules by interstitial fibrosis. The cysts have an atypical hyperplastic epithelial lining that can undergo malignant change.

Simple cysts

These are very common, with incidence increasing with age. They vary in size (usually 2–5 cm in diameter) and number, and contain clear fluid. Microscopically, they have a cuboidal epithelial lining and a thin capsule. Renal function is not affected but pain might be felt if there is haemorrhage into the cyst. The cysts can be differentiated from tumours by ultrasound.

Acute kidney injury and chronic kidney disease

Objectives

By the end of the chapter you should be able to:
- Classify the causes of acute kidney injury (AKI)
- Differentiate prerenal and intrinsic renal AKI
- Describe the common causes of chronic kidney disease (CKD)
- State the stages of CKD
- Predict the complications of CKD
- Understand the dietary management of CKD
- Give five indications for renal replacement therapy
- Explain how haemodialysis works
- Give the benefits and disadvantages of peritoneal dialysis compared to haemodialysis
- State the complications of renal transplantation

TERMINOLOGY

Acute kidney injury (AKI) and chronic kidney disease (CKD) are now the preferred terms for what often used to be described as acute or chronic renal failure, respectively. Renal failure implies reduced excretory function of the kidney whereas CKD can be present even when excretory function is normal, as long as there is other evidence of kidney damage (for example blood or protein in the urine or structural abnormality).

Uraemia

'Uraemia' is the term given to the clinical symptoms which arise when nitrogenous metabolic waste products accumulate in the blood (i.e. urea and creatinine), as a result of decreased filtration of these products by the kidneys. Uraemia may affect any of the body's systems.

ACUTE KIDNEY INJURY

Acute kidney injury is the deterioration of renal function occurring over hours or days. Urea and creatinine rise rapidly. It is usually (but not always) associated with oliguria and is usually (but not always) reversible. The dangerous consequences are volume overload, metabolic acidosis and hyperkalaemia. The causes are classified as shown Fig. 7.1.

Prerenal causes of AKI:

- Reduced effective circulating volume – hypovolaemia (e.g. haemorrhage, dehydration, burns) cardiac failure or liver failure

- Shock (may also lead on to acute tubular necrosis)
- Renal artery stenosis or emboli
- NSAIDs and ACE inhibitors impair the mechanisms of renal autoregulation so can predispose to prerenal AKI.

Intrinsic renal causes of AKI:

- Acute tubular necrosis: ischaemia (can be caused by any prerenal cause), drug toxicity (e.g. gentamicin, aciclovir, methotrexate) and toxins (e.g. myoglobinuria and lipopolysaccharide in Gram-negative sepsis)
- Acute interstitial nephritis (due to drugs, infections, hypercalcaemia, multiple myeloma)
- Glomerular disease – acute glomerulonephritis, rapidly progressive glomerulonephritis
- Vascular disease – vasculitis, malignant hypertension, thrombotic microangiopathies.

Postrenal causes of AKI are:

- Bladder outflow obstruction (benign prostatic hypertrophy or urethral strictures)
- Tumour (prostate, bladder or gynaecological malignancy)
- Stone (would need to be bilateral to cause renal failure)
- Retroperitoneal fibrosis causing ureteral obstruction.

Note: Obstruction must occur in both kidneys or in a single functioning kidney for renal failure to occur.

Diagnostic approach to AKI

First it is important to ask:

- *Is the renal failure acute or chronic?* A history of chronic ill health or signs of CKD such as anaemia may indicate chronicity, as does small kidneys on ultrasound

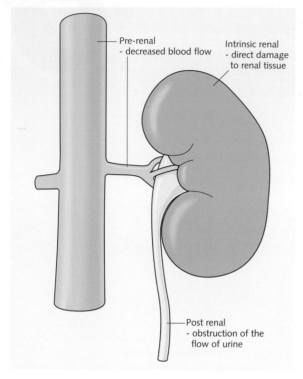

Fig. 7.1 Causes of acute kidney injury. AKI can be caused by decreased blood flow (prerenal), direct damage to the renal tissue (intrinsic renal) or obstruction of the flow of urine (post-renal).

- *Is there urinary tract obstruction?* Obstruction should always be considered as a cause because it is reversible and prompt treatment may prevent permanent renal damage
- *Is there a rare cause of acute kidney injury?* For example, myeloma, systemic vasculitis, haemolytic uraemic syndrome because prompt treatment can be lifesaving.

Basic investigation of acute kidney injury includes urine tests (dipstick, microscopy, culture, cytology), blood tests and renal imaging (KUB (X-ray of the kidney, ureter and bladder), a chest X-ray and an ultrasound of the renal tract). In AKI, the following biochemical changes occur:

- Increased plasma urea and creatinine concentrations
- Increased plasma urate
- Increased plasma concentrations of potassium
- Metabolic acidosis and an increased anion gap
- Increased plasma phosphate and decreased plasma calcium (less marked than in CKD)
- Decreased plasma sodium can occur
- Changes in urine biochemistry: these depend on whether prerenal or renal failure exists (Fig. 7.2).

In addition, some serological tests can help clarify the diagnosis:

- Antinuclear antibodies (ANA): SLE-associated nephritis

Fig. 7.2 Urine biochemistry results.

Test	Prerenal	Intrinsic renal (acute tubular necrosis)
Urine osmolality (mOsm/kg H_2O)	>500	<350
Urine sodium (mmol/L)	<20	>40
Urine/serum creatinine	>40	<20
Urine/serum osmolality	>1.5	<1.2
Fractional excreted sodium	<1	>1
Renal failure index	↑ urea >creatinine	↑ urea ↑ creatinine

- Cryoglobulin titre: cryoglobulinaemia
- Complement levels: SLE-associated nephritis, membranoproliferative and acute glomerulonephritis
- Antineutrophil cytoplasmic antibodies (ANCA): vasculitis (Wegener's granulomatosis or polyangiitis).

Fig. 7.3 gives some clues to help in the diagnosis of acute kidney injury and its possible causes.

Management

Management depends on the precipitating cause.

Appropriate fluid replacement therapy is always important to optimize blood flow to the kidneys. Hypovolaemia is a common cause of prerenal failure and will lead to acute tubular necrosis if left uncorrected. Hypovolaemia should be rapidly corrected with intravenous fluids. Clinical signs of dehydration include, decreased skin turgor, a low JVP, a low blood pressure, weight loss. Invasive monitoring of the central venous pressure may be necessary to confirm hypovolaemia.

Obstruction of bladder outflow is relieved with a urinary or suprapubic catheter. If the ureters are obstructed, a drainage tube (nephrostomy) is inserted above the obstruction.

Clinical Note

Life-threatening complications of AKI include hyperkalaemia, pulmonary oedema and bleeding. They need urgent treatment and renal replacement therapy may be needed.

CHRONIC KIDNEY DISEASE

CKD can result in progressive loss of renal function over months to years. It is usually irreversible because the renal tissue has been replaced by extracellular matrix (scar tissue) in response to damage. However, the

Fig. 7.3 Clues to help in diagnosis of acute kidney injury and its possible causes.

	Prerenal	Intrinsic renal	Postrenal
History	Thirst; weight loss; potential for volume loss (e.g. surgery, diuretics); ineffective circulating volume	Previous abnormal urinalysis; exposure to toxic agents; hypertension; new medications	Frequency; hesitancy; nocturia; history of nephrolithiasis or neoplasms; renal colic especially if only one kidney
Physical examination	Signs of dehydration: hypotension; hypovolaemia; ↓ BP = postural drop; ↑ pulse; ↓ jugular venous pulse	Hypertension; physical signs (e.g. skin lesions of vasculitis)	Distended bladder; enlarged prostate
Urinalysis	↑ Urine osmolality and high specific gravity; ↓ urine Na^+ and fractional excreted Na^+; ↑ urine:serum creatinine	Proteinuria; haematuria; pyuria; renal tubular epithelial cells in urinary sediment; casts and their nature	Crystalluria (suggests renal calculus)

Fig. 7.4 Classification of chronic kidney disease according to estimated glomerular filtration rate (eGFR).

Stage	eGFR	Description
1	>90	Kidney damage with normal or increased eGFR
2	60–89	Kidney damage with mild eGFR fall
3A	45–59	Moderate fall in eGFR
3B	30–44	
4	15–29	Severe fall in eGFR
5	<15	Established renal failure

Note: To diagnose stages 1–2 there must also be (non-urological) haematuria or proteinuria or a known renal structural abnormality.

deterioration can be slowed with treatment. It can result from renal disease or be secondary to systemic diseases.

Progression of CKD is best monitored by plotting the calculated or estimated glomerular filtration rate (see Chapter 2) against time (Fig. 7.4). At first there may be no symptoms, only biochemical abnormalities but in later stages symptoms develop from the loss of excretory, endocrine and metabolic functions. It is likely that renal replacement therapy will be needed by stage 5. The rate of death from cardiovascular disease is greatly increased in CKD especially stages 4 and 5.

Screening of people at risk

NICE have recommended that people in the following at risk groups should be offered testing for CKD:

- Diabetes
- Hypertension
- Cardiovascular disease (ischaemic heart disease, chronic heart failure, peripheral vascular disease and cerebral vascular disease)
- Structural renal tract disease, renal calculi or prostatic hypertrophy

- Multisystem diseases with potential kidney involvement, e.g. systemic lupus erythematosus (SLE)
- Family history of stage 5 CKD or hereditary kidney disease
- Patients on known nephrotxic drugs
- Opportunistic detection of haematuria or proteinuria.

Annual follow-up testing is recommended in all patients with CKD or at risk of CKD, with more frequent testing being required according to clinical circumstance or during an intercurrent illness.

Causes

Causes of CKD are:

- **Intrinsic renal**: glomerulonephritis, chronic pyelonephritis, polycystic kidneys, bladder or urethral obstruction, interstitial nephritis, amyloid, myeloma, renal vascular disease, Alport's syndrome
- **Systemic (extrarenal)**: diabetes mellitus, hypertension (especially if accelerated-malignant), heart failure, SLE, gout, hypercalcaemia, renovascular disease (atheroma), vasculitis
- **Drugs**: gold, penicillamine, ciclosporin, analgesics.

> **HINTS AND TIPS**
>
> The commonest causes of CKD are diabetes, hypertension, reflux nephropathy and polycystic kidney disease.

The diagnostic approach to CKD can involve:

- **Urine**: urinalysis (haematuria, proteinuria), microscopy (white cells, eosinophilia, granular casts, red cell casts, red cells), biochemistry (protein or albumin to creatinine ration, urinary electrolytes, osmolality, protein electrophoresis)
- **Blood**: urea and creatinine and eGFR, electrolytes, glucose, calcium (decreased), phosphate (increased), urate (increased), protein, osmolality, full blood count, markers of inflammation (C-reactive protein (CRP) or erythrocyte sedimentation rate (ESR)), protein electrophoresis, autoantibody screen, complement components
- **Radiology**: ultrasound (to assess the kidney size, identify obstruction, mass lesions or polycystic kidney disease). Plain radiography or CT of the abdomen (calculi) and chest X-ray (pulmonary oedema). Hand radiographs can show evidence of osteodystrophy in advanced cases but are now rarely performed
- **Renal biopsy**: consider if kidneys are of normal size and the cause of CKD is not clear from other investigations.

Preventing progression of CKD

Damage which has resulted in CKD cannot be reversed but it is important to effectively treat any cause to prevent further damage, for example relieving any obstruction of urine flow or stopping any nephrotoxic drugs. Hypertension must be effectively treated and this may require several antihypertensives. Diabetics need tight control of their blood glucose and benefit from ACE inhibitors or ARBs, as do patients with proteinuria. The presence of proteinuria is a poor prognostic sign.

Protein restriction to prevent progression of CKD is now rarely recommended as it is likely to cause malnutrition.

Complications and management

Fluid retention

This can cause pulmonary oedema or peripheral oedema. Treatment is with diuretics which are less effective in renal failure so bigger doses may be needed.

Hypertension

This can be caused by CKD and is an important cause of progression in CKD. It must therefore be carefully treated. Drugs which interfere with the renin–angiotensin system may be particularly effective if they can be tolerated. The targets for treatment are shown in Fig. 7.5.

Increased cardiovascular risk

This is another reason to tightly control blood pressure. Other cardiovascular risk factors must also be addressed and many patients will benefit from lifestyle advice, aspirin and a statin.

Osteodystrophy

In advanced CKD failure to activate vitamin D leads to hypocalcaemia and impaired mineralization of bone. Also the kidneys do not excrete enough phosphate. This stimulates PTH release which increases bone reabsorption. Bone pains are experienced in the lower back and legs. Treatment is with vitamin D analogues, calcium supplements, reducing phosphate intake in the diet and reducing phosphate absorption with phosphate-binding agents.

Fig. 7.5 Blood pressure targets in CKD.	
Target	**Condition**
120–139/90	Non-diabetic CKD
120–129/80	CKD with proteinuria or diabetes

Anaemia

In advanced CKD there is reduced erythropoietin production by the kidney. In addition retained toxins reduced red blood cell survival and impair bone marrow responsiveness to erythropoietin. This leads to a normocytic normochromic anaemia. Symptoms are lethargy and dyspnoea. Anaemia of CKD can be effectively reversed by (expensive) erythropoietin injections, but it is essential to ensure iron stores are adequate prior to starting treatment.

Electrolyte disturbances

Some electrolyte imbalances can be managed with dietary changes (Fig. 7.6).

Fig. 7.6 Dietary changes in chronic kidney disease.

Disturbance	Dietary treatment
Fluid retention	Sodium and fluid restriction
Hyperphosphataemia	Phosphate restriction, phosphate-binding agents
Hypekalaemia	Potassium restriction
Hypocalcaemia	Calcium and vitamin D supplements

Acidosis

Metabolic acidosis can be treated with sodium bicarbonate or calcium carbonate supplements.

Uraemia

Inability to excrete nitrogenous waste products can lead to uraemic symptoms. This may include anorexia, nausea and vomiting. Itching is also a common complaint (this is also caused by hyperphosphataemia). When advanced uraemia can cause neuromuscular symptoms (restless legs and fitting). The only effective treatment for uraemic symptoms is renal replacement therapy.

RENAL REPLACEMENT THERAPY

In end-stage kidney disease it is necessary to replace the excretory function of the kidneys with renal replacement therapy (RRT). The four forms of RRT are: haemodialysis, haemofiltration, peritoneal dialysis and renal transplantation (Fig. 7.7). These remove the waste products and excess fluids that accumulate in renal disease, but only renal transplantation can replace all the kidney's functions.

In CKD the indications for RRT are not clear cut and the onset should be planned in accordance with the

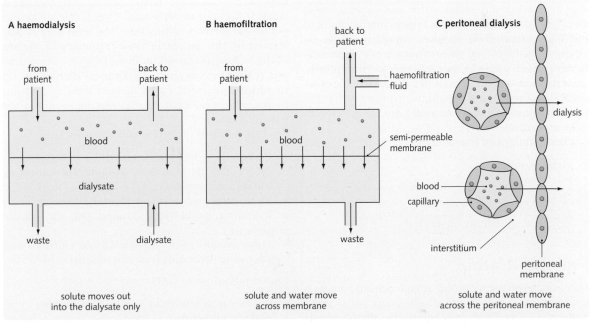

Fig. 7.7 Comparison of the three different methods of dialysis. (A) haemodialysis; (B) haemofiltration and (C) peritoneal dialysis. (Adapted from O'Callaghan CA, Bremmer BM, 2001. The kidney at a glance. Blackwell Science, pp. 96, 98.)

patient's symptoms and eGFR. The indications for RRT in AKI include:

- Hyperkalaemia
- Pulmonary oedema
- Acidosis
- Uraemic pericarditis.

Haemodialysis

This involves using a dialysis machine to pump blood through an artificial kidney. Blood flows on one side of a semipermeable membrane, with dialysis fluid being passed in the opposite direction on the other side. Dialysis occurs across the semipermeable membrane removing toxins from the blood down a concentration gradient.

The dialysate is made of purified water with a solute composition similar to plasma, but without any of the waste products, so solutes move along their concentration gradient out of the blood. Smaller solutes diffuse across the semipermeable membrane faster than larger solutes. Dialysis 'dose' can be adjusted by altering the blood flow, the area of the semipermeable membrane, or the duration of treatment. On average, patients require at least 4 hours of treatment three times a week. Coagulation within the dialysis machine is prevented with heparin. Treatment may be performed in a hospital environment supervised by a nursing team or at home by the patient themselves after a period of training.

Access to the circulation is gained by an arteriovenous (AV) fistula, which is constructed surgically, usually by joining the radial artery and cephalic vein. Over a few weeks the venous system 'arterializes' and the high blood flow required for dialysis can be obtained by 'needling' the venous system. Complications of the AV fistula include infection and thrombosis. A fistula should be prepared well in advance of the onset of RRT. If a fistula is not possible then quick access to the circulation can be gained through a double lumen central venous catheter.

Complications of haemodialysis include:

- Hypotension
- Infection
- Haemolysis
- Air embolism
- Reactions to dialysis membrane.

Haemofiltration

This involves filtering blood at high pressure across a semipermeable membrane allowing removal of small molecules. The fluid lost across the membrane is discarded and replacement with an appropriate biochemical composition is added back to the blood. This replacement fluid is commonly buffered by lactate.

Haemofiltration is used predominantly for the treatment of AKI, especially in the intensive care unit setting. When performed slowly (continuous veno–veno haemofiltration), it causes smaller fluid shifts and therefore less hypotension than haemodialysis. Access is obtained through a double lumen central venous catheter. Haemodiafiltration is a combination of dialysis and filtration through the same machine.

Peritoneal dialysis

This is usually undertaken using continuous ambulatory peritoneal dialysis (CAPD). CAPD uses the peritoneal membrane as the semipermeable membrane. Unlike haemodialysis, peritoneal dialysis does not require an AV fistula for circulatory access. Instead, it requires the insertion of a permanent 'Tenchkoff' catheter through the anterior abdominal wall into the peritoneal cavity. Dialysate solution is introduced into the peritoneum and exchanged regularly for fresh fluid – up to four or five times a day is necessary to maintain the efficiency of dialysis. Waste products pass into the dialysate along their concentration gradients and water is removed by osmosis. Dialysis solutions with high osmolarity will remove more water. Dextrose is the most commonly used osmotic agent, but is gradually absorbed by the patient. Newer, nonabsorbable, osmotic agents are now available (e.g. glucose polymer). CAPD is used in the maintenance dialysis of end-stage renal failure, but technique survival declines to 50% after 5 years due to loss of peritoneal membrane function. The treatment is performed by the patient in the community. A variant of the technique is continuous cycling peritoneal dialysis (CCPD) or automated peritoneal dialysis (APD) in which a machine cycles dialysis fluid in and out of the peritoneal cavity, usually at night whilst the patient is asleep.

Complications of peritoneal dialysis include:

- Peritonitis (50% is caused by *Staphylococcus epidermidis*). Treatment is with intraperitoneal or intravenous antibiotics
- Mechanical problems with fluid drainage
- Infections or blockage around the site of the catheter
- Other complications include pleural effusions and sclerosing peritonitis (rare but serious).

Contraindications to CAPD are:

- Peritoneal adhesions as a result of peritonitis
- Abdominal hernia
- Colostomy
- Less effective in obese patients.

Renal transplantation

This is the ideal treatment for irreversible stage 5 CKD. It restores near-normal renal function and improves quality of life. The kidney may come from a cadaver, a close living relative or a partner and is usually placed in the iliac fossa. The renal vessels from the donated kidney are anastomosed onto the iliac blood vessels of the recipient and the ureter is inserted into the bladder (Fig. 7.8). Success depends upon:

* ABO group
* HLA types
* Immunosuppressive treatment.

Short-term complications include:

* Acute rejection (within 3 months)
* Operative failure.

The risk of rejection is reduced by immunosuppression therapy, which is started at the time of the transplant and continued indefinitely. The patients are at risk of opportunistic infection (e.g. with cytomegalovirus).
Long-term complications include:

* Infection
* Recurrence of original disease

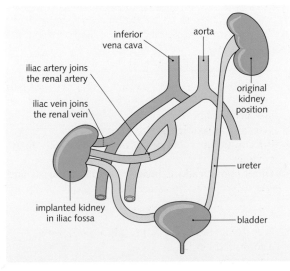

* Obstruction at the ureteric anastomoses
* Malignancy, especially lymphomas.

Currently, the 1-year graft survival rate is in excess of 80% for cadaveric transplants and 90% for live donor transplants.

PHARMACOKINETICS IN RENAL DISEASE

There are many factors to think about when prescribing drugs for a patient with kidney disease. Nephrotoxic drugs need to be avoided and the pharmacokinetics of other drugs can be changed.

Absorption

Fluid retention in kidney disease with oedema of the bowel wall can lead to reduced absorption of drugs given orally.

Distribution

The protein binding of drugs may be affected in proteinuric renal disease because of hypoalbuminaemia. Also, with uraemia other retained substances compete for binding sites of the drug. This will increase the concentration of the drug in the blood. Fluid retention in kidney disease can increase the volume of distribution.

Metabolism

The kidney metabolizes some drugs, e.g. insulin. If this function is impaired the half life of the drug will increase. Uraemia can also alter drug metabolism by the liver.

Elimination

Excretion of drugs by the kidney is a major route of elimination. If this function of the kidney is impaired the half life of the drug will be increased and the plasma concentration will rise with each dose of the drug. Renal elimination is particularly important with water-soluble drugs that are minimally metabolized by the liver.

Fig. 7.8 Implantation of a transplanted kidney.

● **Objectives**

By the end of the chapter you should be able to:
- List the symptoms typically relevant to the urinary system
- Explain why family history is sometimes important in kidney disease
- Find relevant signs in a patient's hands
- Describe how to measure the jugular venous pulse
- Differentiate an enlarged kidney from splenomegaly
- Describe the test for ascites and the renal causes of it
- Name five tests that can be performed on a urine sample, and explain the importance of a mid-stream urine sample
- List the causes of haematuria and proteinuria and explain how they might be investigated
- List the blood tests that can be done to investigate renal function, and give the possible causes of abnormal results
- Explain when you would use ultrasonography in preference to plain radiography
- List the contraindications for renal biopsy, and four potential complications
- Describe the complications of using intravenous contrast medium
- Explain the main differences between a diagnostic and a therapeutic cystoscopy
- Explain how urodynamics studies can be used to differentiate between genuine stress incontinence and urge incontinence

HISTORY

This section is a guide to taking a history for the renal and urinary systems. Not all will be relevant to each patient and you may need to inquire about other systems to investigate a differential diagnosis.

History of presenting complaint

Fig. 8.1 shows typical symptoms of diseases of the urinary system. As always, enquire deeper about the presenting complaint. Use open questions and non-verbal prompting where possible. Use the mnemonics SQITARS (Site, Quality, Intensity, Timing, Aggravating factors, Relieving factors, and associated Symptoms) or SOCRATES (Site, Onset, Character, Radiation, Associated symptoms, Timing, Exacerbating and alleviating factors, Severity) to help you to gather as much information as possible.

Past medical history

Find out any past or current medical illnesses, operations or trauma. Past history of any renal or urological disease is obviously important. Diabetes and hypertension are risk factors for CKD. Systemic diseases such as vasculitis can cause glomerulonephritis. CKD is related to a higher risk of cardiovascular disease. A recent streptococcal throat infection can trigger post-streptococcal glomerulonephritis.

Drug history

Find out all the medications that the patient takes. Also ask about over-the-counter medicine and homeopathic medicine. Many medications can affect renal function (Fig. 8.2). Also remember that the pharmacokinetics of drugs can be altered in renal disease.

Family history

Polycystic kidney disease, Alport's syndrome and Fabry's syndrome are inherited renal diseases. Many other diseases will have some genetic component. A family history of CKD stage 5 increases the risk of an individual having CKD. Some families have a tendency for IgA nephropathy. Also ask about family history of diabetes and hypertension. Ethnicity is important in the incidence of some diseases, e.g. SLE and diabetic nephropathy in South Asian populations.

Fig 8.1 Symptoms of the renal and urinary systems.

Renal symptoms	Loin pain, oedema, oliguria, anuria, polyuria, nocturia, frank haematuria
Uraemic symptoms	Lethargy, fatigue, anorexia, pruritus, bone pain, nausea, vomiting
Lower urinary tract symptoms:	Urgency, frequency, dysuria, incontinence, hesitancy, dribbling, suprapubic pain, haematuria

Fig 8.2 Drugs that can impair renal function.

Drug	Nephrotoxicity
ACE inhibitors, angiotensin receptor Blockers	Exacerbate prerenal AKI
NSAIDs	Exacerbate prerenal AKI, tubulointerstitial nephritis
Gold, penicillamine	Membranous glomerulonephritis
Aminoglycosides, radio-opaque contrast, amphotericin B, furosemide, cephalosporins	Acute tubular necrosis
Lithium, cyclosporin, tacrolimus, penicillins	Tubulointerstitial nephritis

Social history

A patient's social situation can be very important in deciding management. Ask about their marital status, social support network, hobbies and how they are coping at work. Other factors in the social history:

- Occupation. Has the patient been exposed to any toxins? Workers in rubber and dye factories can be exposed to aromatic amines that can cause bladder cancer
- Smoking is a risk factor for bladder cancer and renal vascular disease
- Alcohol can compromise kidney function
- Dietary habits can be relevant in urolithiasis (calcium, oxalate and fluid intake) and CKD (protein, fluid, sodium, phosphate, iron intake)
- Sexual history may be relevant if there is a possibility of STI.

HINTS AND TIPS

- Use open questions to establish the patient's beliefs
- Use closed questions to obtain and classify facts to narrow down the patient's diagnosis.

Ideas, concerns and expectations

It is important to find out patient's ideas and concerns regarding their presentation. Ask what they are hoping the doctor can do for them; this may seem obvious but different patients bring different agendas and this will affect your management later.

EXAMINATION

General inspection

Whenever you examine a patient it is important to remember the following points:

- Introduce yourself to the patient and ask permission to examine them
- Position the patient appropriately for the examination – at 45° for cardiovascular or respiratory system examination or lying flat for abdominal examination
- Expose the appropriate part of the body only and ensure the patient is comfortable
- Observe the patient carefully from the end of the bed before you begin the examination
- Look around the patient for any extra clues – dialysis equipment, sputum pot or oxygen mask
- Notice if the patient is conscious or looks well, is in pain, appears anxious or depressed, smells of urine or has any obvious skeletal abnormalities
- Look at the patient's stature (CKD in childhood causes growth retardation)
- Weighing the patient regularly can be helpful if they are retaining fluid.

Hands

Abnormalities of the nails that indicate underlying renal disease are summarized in Fig. 8.3. To examine the hands, spread out the fingers on a flat, white surface. This will highlight any shortening of the distal phalanges; a difference of length between the fingers is often seen in severe renal osteodystrophy secondary to chronic renal failure. This is due to chronic high circulating levels of parathyroid hormone. With the patient holding their hands straight out, look for a course flapping movement called asterexis. Whilst this could be caused by severe uraemia it cannot be distinguished from asterexis caused by CO_2 retention or liver failure.

Pinch the skin on the back of the hand to determine its elasticity or turgor. Reduced skin turgor can be caused by old age but can also indicate dehydration.

Fig 8.3 Nail signs in renal disease.

Test	Sign	Diagnostic inference
Look for markings on nail	Splinter haemorrhages	Renal disease due to: • Vasculitis (e.g. Wegener's granulomatosis) • Bacterial endocarditis
	Transverse ridges (Beau's lines)	Indicative of: • Past malnutrition • Severe illness
Look for discoloration of nails	Brown discoloration of nails	Chronic kidney disease
	White nails (leukonychia)	Hypoalbuminaemia, e.g. from nephrotic syndrome

Arms

Look in the arms for an arteriovenous fistula, used for dialysis access. If you find a fistula:

• Palpate it to check it has a thrill
• Auscultate over it to check it has a good bruit.

Bruising can occur in uraemia as can scratch marks associated with pruritus.

Blood pressure

This is very important in renal disease. When measuring blood pressure (which needs to be done on several occasions) it is important to measure it on the same limb each time to ensure consistent and comparable results. To ensure measurement is accurate:

• Select the correct cuff size
• Use the cuff on a fully extended arm with the stethoscope applied lightly to the brachial artery
• Always take the blood pressure with the patient sitting and standing. This is because a 5–10 mmHg increase in diastolic pressure is usually seen on standing in a patient with a healthy cardiovascular system (CVS). Postural hypotension (i.e. a drop in diastolic pressure on standing) can be detected only if both measurements are made.

The World Health Organization (WHO) defines hypertension as maintained systolic pressure of 140 mmHg or above and a diastolic pressure of 90 mmHg or above. However, blood pressure levels lower than this are associated with improved survival in epidemiological studies. Most renal diseases are associated with the development of hypertension.

Face

In the face you will want to check the general appearance, look at the conjunctivae for pallor and look in the mouth for ulcers, infections and fetor. You may want to carry out ophthalmoscopy and check the patient's hearing. The facial signs related to renal disease are listed in Fig. 8.4.

Neck

Identify any central venous lines placed that may be used for dialysis access.

Measure the jugular venous pressure (JVP) which is a good indicator of fluid load. The patient should be at 45° and with the head turned to the left. Look between the two heads of the sternocleidomastoid on the left side and note any pulsations in the internal jugular vein. This can be differentiated from visible arterial pulsations because:

• There are two pulsations per heartbeat (in sinus rhythm)
• The predominant movement is inward
• It rises with abdominal pressure or expiration.

If a waveform is visible then measure the height from the top of the fluid level vertically down to the angle of Louis. More than 4 cm is considered raised.

Clinical Note

A raised JVP indicates:
• Fluid overload
• Right heart failure
• COPD – cor pulmonale.

Thorax

Observe the shape of the chest which can be deformed by renal osteodystrophy (a late sign).

Respiratory system

Few signs in a respiratory examination indicate renal disease. A key change to watch for is the pattern and rate

Fig 8.4 Signs in the face related to renal disease.

Test	Sign	Diagnostic inference
General appearance	Red and rugged appearance of the face	Sign of polycythaemia occasionally seen in: • Polycystic kidneys • Post-transplant • Carcinoma of the kidney
Pull down the eyelid and look at conjunctiva	Pale conjunctiva	Anaemia can be caused by CKD
Look for deposits on forehead	White powdery crystals of urate look like dandruff on the forehead	Sign of uraemic frost – the crystals form from excess urea in the sweat and are a preterminal sign of CKD
Look for deposits in the sclera	Yellow deposits in the sclera	Calcium deposits due to hyperparathyroidism
Look for retinal changes	Retinal changes typical of diabetes, hypertension and vascular disease	Seen in: • Diabetes mellitus • Hypertension • Vascular disease
Check hearing	Deafness	Alport syndrome
Look at mucous membranes of mouth	White deposit in the mouth of fungal infection	Patients on cytotoxic drugs or steroids; immunosuppression with drugs can result in opportunistic infections such as candidal infection
Be aware of patients's breath	Halitosis (bad breath), either: • Ammonia smell • Acetone smell	Respectively due to: • Renal failure • Ketoacidosis

CKD, chronic kidney disease

of respiration – patients with a metabolic acidosis associated with chronic kidney disease often have a deep, sigh-like respiration, with a rapid breathing rate. This is known as Kussmaul's respiration, and is caused by direct stimulation of the respiratory centre in an attempt to correct the systemic acidosis.

Bilateral pleural effusions can occur in nephrotic syndrome or fluid overload. The signs are dullness to percussion, reduced breath sounds and reduced vocal resonance.

Listen for fine inspiratory crackles indicating pulmonary oedema. This can be caused by volume overload causing congestive cardiac failure.

Cardiovascular system

The kidneys are linked to the cardiovascular examination because volume overload, hypertension and anaemia can produce cardiovascular signs. Palpate the apex beat which might be laterally displaced in left ventricular dilatation, thrusting in hypertension and left ventricular hypertrophy.

Auscultate the heart sounds listening particularly for:

- Low-pitched third or fourth heart sounds, associated with fluid overload or left ventricular failure
- Pericardial rub, a scratching sound heard in any part of the cardiac sound with the patient leaning forwards. It can be caused by uraemic pericarditis.

Abdomen

The patient should be lying as flat as possible on a firm mattress with arms by the side and head supported with one or two pillows – check that the patient is comfortable. This position ensures that the abdominal muscles are relaxed, making palpation much easier.

Stand on the right-hand side of the bed, ideally with the patient exposed from 'nipples to knees'; to maintain privacy expose the patient from the xiphisternum to the level of the symphysis pubis.

Inspection

Spend the first 20–30 s inspecting the patient from the end of the bed. Look around the patient for any clues – drips, drains and dialysis machines. Fig. 8.5 gives the signs usually seen on general inspection of the abdomen in a patient with renal disease.

Palpation

Before palpating, check if the patient is in pain. If the answer is yes, ask where the painful or tender area is and start palpating from the point furthest from the locus of the pain. Tell the patient to breathe normally and relax – you will be able to feel much more through relaxed abdominal muscles. It can help to kneel at the bedside so that you are at the same level as the patient – always demonstrate this in an examination.

Develop a routine for examining all the regions and organs to avoid omitting anything:

- Begin with gentle palpation of the nine regions of the abdomen; then repeat using deeper palpation – keep looking at the patient's face for any signs of discomfort
- Feel for the liver and spleen while the patient is breathing deeply in and out
- Next examine the kidneys and urinary bladder, feeling for the aorta, and then check the hernial

orifices (inguinal and femoral) while the patient is coughing
- If you feel a mass, define its site, size, shape, edge, surface (regular or irregular), consistency, mobility, movement with respiration and whether it is pulsatile or resonant to percussion. Also check for associated scars and listen over the mass for a bruit.

Fig. 8.6 explains how the kidneys are examined and gives the relevant findings in various renal conditions. The differentiating features between an enlarged left kidney and splenomegaly are summarized in Fig. 8.7.

Clinical Note

The kidneys are usually not palpable except in very thin people. When they are enlarged, however, be careful, because an enlarged kidney can easily be confused with:
- Hepatomegaly (right)
- Splenomegaly (left).

Percussion

Percussion in the abdomen is used to elicit the cause of any distension and the composition of any mass – fluid-filled cysts and solid tumours are dull on percussion. The

Fig. 8.5 Findings on general inspection of the abdomen in renal disease.

Test	Sign	Diagnostic inference
Look for abnormality of the abdominal contours:		Renal causes of a distended abdomen are: • Fluid (ascites or CAPD fluid)
• General distension	• General fullness and enlargement of the abdominal cavity • The skin of the abdomen is shiny and smooth	Other (non-renal) causes include: • Fat • Flatus • Fetus • Faeces (constipation)
• Localized distension: observe to see if abdomen moves with or independently of respiration	Symmetrical swelling	Polycystic kidneys
	Asymmetrical swelling	Enlarged kidney; kidney transplant in the iliac regions
Look for scars: note position on the abdomen and check round to the back following the ribs to the spine	Midline scars	Previous abdominal surgery
	Iliac scars overlying a mass	Kidney transplant
	lateral longitudinal scars extending around the back	Nephrectomy scars
	Note that old scars are white and pale and recent scars are purple-red in colour	

CAPD, continuous ambulatory peritoneal dialysis.

Fig. 8.6 How to examine the kidneys and relevant findings in a variety of renal conditions.

Test	Sign	Diagnostic inference
Bimanual examination of the kidneys (balloting): • Place the right hand anteriorly in the lumbar region and the left hand posteriorly under the patient in the loin • Push up with the left hand as the patient takes a deep breath in • Ballot the kidneys between both hands (i.e. push the kidney from one hand to the other) • Repeat on the other side keeping the right hand anterior	The kidney is normally impalpable (except in very thin people) and if easily felt suggests an abnormality The lower pole is felt as a firm round edge between both hands on deep inspiration (it must be distinguished from an enlarged liver or spleen) There is minimal movement on respiration An irregular kidney surface felt in polycystic disease	Unilateral enlargement: • Tumour • Renal cyst • Hydronephrosis • Compensatory hypertrophy Bilateral enlargement: • Polycystic kidneys • Hydronephrosis • Tumour (rare)
Examination of the urinary bladder: • The bladder is palpated from the umbilicus down to the symphysis pubis • The upper and lateral borders are easily felt • The inferior border is impalpable	Not normally palpable When enlarged it is felt as a smooth rounded firm cystic mass in the suprabupic region It is not always symmetrical and in the midline	Chronic retention of urine Acute retention is associated with bladder tenderness Distended bladders are not always palpable in obesity
Pain: • Check carefully if the patient is in pain • The nature of the pain is important in determining the site of the lesion • Assess pain by asking the patient to point to the pain and asking what the pain is like	Fixed constant pain; colicky pain superimposed on a constant dull pain	Kidney pain
	Radiation of pain from the flank to the groin and iliac fossa; the patient is usually writhing in pain and is doubled up	Ureteric distension due to obstruction in the ureters, most commonly renal stones as they are passed down the ureter

Fig. 8.7 Features that distinguish between left kidney enlargement and splenomegaly.

Enlarged left kidney	Splenomegaly
Moves late with inspiration	Moves early in inspiration
Can feel above it	Cannot get above it; enlarges towards the umbilicus
Smooth surface	Notched border palpable
Resonant to percussion	Dull to percussion

HINTS AND TIPS

Remember the causes of a distended abdomen as the '5 Fs':
- Fat
- Fluid
- Flatus
- Fetus
- Faeces.

presence of ascites (excess free fluid in the peritoneal cavity) is shown by shifting dullness. To examine for this the abdomen is percussed from the midline into the flank for any areas of dullness. Keep your finger on the area of dullness whilst asking the patient to roll away from you on to their side. Percuss this area with the patient in the new position and see if it is now resonant to percussion. This is due to redistribution of fluid in the peritoneal cavity.

The causes of ascites in renal disease are:

- Nephrotic syndrome
- Peritoneal dialysis fluid
- Idiopathic ascites of dialysis.

Auscultation

A bruit is heard if there is rapid turbulent movement of blood through a narrowed artery. Causes of renal bruits include:

- Renal artery stenosis
- Atherosclerosis
- Arteriovenous malformation in the kidney.

Renal bruits can be heard by auscultating just superior to the umbilicus or in the flank. However, it can be difficult to distinguish a renal bruit from one originating in the aorta.

Digital rectal examination

Always obtain permission and have a chaperone. The patient should lie on the left side, with the knees drawn up to the chest.

- Inspect the perianal area for haemorrhoids, fissures, inflammation, prolapse and ulcers
- Put lubricant on the glove and insert finger into the rectum
- Assess the tone of the anal sphincter and the size and shape of the prostate (normally walnut-sized)
- After removing your finger, inspect for any blood or faeces.

Palpable changes in the prostate and their clinical significance are summarized in Fig. 8.8. A vaginal examination should also be performed in female patients. (See *Crash Course: Obstetrics and Gynaecology* for further details.)

Legs

Examine the legs for rashes which might indicate vasculitis related to the kidneys, e.g. Henoch-Schönlein purpura.

If the legs are swollen confirm that it is pitting oedema by pressing for a few seconds and seeing if the indentation remains afterwards. This is associated with nephrotic syndrome and volume overload.

TESTING THE BLOOD AND URINE

Diseases of the renal and urinary tract are suggested by symptoms linked to the urinary tract, abnormal urinalysis or abnormal serum urea or creatinine concentration. Testing the urine is the simplest investigation and should always be done in suspected renal disease. This is done with a midstream urine (MSU) sample, and assessment includes appearance, pH, dipstick, microscopy and cytological examination (Figs 8.9 and 8.10).

Fig. 8.8 Changes of the prostate noted on digital rectal examination.

Sign	Diagnostic inference
Firm, smooth, rubbery consistency; walnut-shaped and sized	Normal prostate
Tender, enlarged and soft	Acute infection (prostatitis)
Hard, irregular, asymmetric, nodular	Prostate carcinoma

Fig. 8.9 Microbiological tests and their significance.

	Indications	Scientific basis	Normal results	Abnormal results
Urine culture	Must always be performed if UTI symptoms or any renal disease is suspected; in cases of TB an early morning sample of urine is required	Growing any organisms present; vital to have an MSU specimen	No growth	>100 000 CFU/mL indicates urinary infection; <10 000 CFU/mL probably indicates contamination of the specimen
Antibodies **(i) Streptococcal Ag**	Suspicion of past streptococcal glomerulonephritis	Antibodies are made in response to infection and may trigger glomerulonephritis		Increased titres of: Anti-DNAase B ASOT Consistent with poststreptococcal glomerulonephritis
(ii) Hepatitis	Renal disease associated with liver disease	Infection with hepatitis B and C has effects on the kidney		Hepatitis B causes: Polyarteritis nodosa; membranous nephropathy Hepatitis C causes: Cryoglobulinaemia
(iii) HIV	Patients at risk of HIV with renal symptoms	Infection with HIV can cause renal damage		HIV-associated glomerulonephritis
malaria	Those who have recently returned from the tropics and have recurrent fevers			Ring-form parasites observed on peripheral blood film

Ag, antigen; ASOT, antistreptococcal O antigen titre; CFU, colony-forming units; HIV, human immunodeficiency virus; MSU, mid-stream urine; TB, tuberculosis; UTI, urinary tract infection.

Fig. 8.10 Urine test results and their significance.

	Indications	Scientific basis	Normal results	Abnormal results
Appearance	Any urine sample		Clear fluid	**Red/pink:** haematuria, beetroot intake **Brown:** concentrated cholestatic jaundice **Cloudy:** infection
Volume	Any urine sample		1000–2500 mL/day	**Oliguria:** physiological; intrinsic renal disease; obstructive nephropathy **Polyuria:** excess H_2O intake; increased solute loss, e.g. glucose; concentration failure
pH	Any urine sample		pH 4.5–8.0	**Alkaline urine:** infection with Proieus–urea splitting **Acid urine:** aminoaciduria; renal calculi
Sodium	Oliguria Altered Na^+ homeostasis	Urinary [Na] must be interpreted in context of urine output, sodium intake and natriuretic drugs	Depends on clinical setting; 24-hour urinary Na^+ = 100–250 mmol/L	<20 mmol/L oliguria aminoaciduria; renal calculi <20 mmol/L oliguria → prerenal <20 mmol/L and not oliguric → extrarenal losses >20 mmol/L renal losses
Creatinine and creatinine clearance	Similar to those for blood creatinine levels	Creatinine clearance reflects GFR; both the urine and plasma concentration of creatinine is required; requires timed urine collection. Now rarely performed	125 mL/min per 1.73 m^2 body surface area	Decreased levels indicate a decrease in GFR–as seen in acute and chronic renal diseases
Blood	Gross bleeding into urine usually found in patients with renal disease; hypertension; pregnancy; bacterial endocarditis	Reagent strips are used – based on a peroxide-like reaction	Nil Any positive result must be followed by microscopy	**Microscopic haematuria:** renal disease, i.e. nephritic syndrome; blood at the beginning of voiding then clear – from the urethra; Blood throughout voiding – from the bladder or above; blood only at the end of voiding – from the prostate or base of the bladder
Protein dipstick and if positive → protein or albumin to creatinine ratio (or 24-hour collection)	Oedema	Reagent strips impregnated with buffered blue tetrabromophenol –detects [albumin] >150 mg/L; microalbuminuria is used as an earlier indicator of diabetic glomerular disease; the test requires a radioimmunoassay ↑ which is more sensitive than the strips	PCR <45 mg/mmol or <150 mg/day (>0.3 g/L is detected on the sticks) microalbuminuria = 0.2–2.8 mg/mmol of creatinine or 30–150 µg/min	**Increased with:** exercise; standing up; renal disease; nephrotic syndrome; fever; diabetic glomerular disease; hypertension
Glucose	Suspected diabetes mellitus; renal disease; pregnancy	Reagent strips using glucose oxidase or hexokinase enzyme reactions Clinitest	Nil	**Glucose may be present when:** 1. Blood glucose above the renal threshold, i.e. diabetes mellitus 2. Altered renal threshold, i.e. pregnancy; renal disease
Urine microscopy (obtain a clean urine sample, i.e. MSU) **(i) Direct** **(ii) After centrifugation**	Symptoms of UTIs; suspicion of renal disease	A small amount of unspun urine placed on a slide, covered with a cover slip and looked at under a microscope Gram stain to look for bacteria Counterstained to look at cytology	Nil	**White cells indicate:** Inflammatory reaction; infection in the urinary tract; stones; TB; analgesic nephropathy **Red cells indicate:** Glomerulonephritis; acute urinary tract infection; calculi; tumour **Granular casts indicate:** Acute tubular necrosis; rapidly progressing glomerulonephritis **White blood cell casts indicate:** Pyelonephritis **Red cell casts indicate:** Glomerulonephritis **Crystals seen indicate:** Stones **Bacteria seen indicate:** Infection **Abnormal cells indicate:** Cancer of urothelium

MSU, mid-stream; TB tuberclosis; UTI, urinary tract infection; GFR, glomerular filtration rate; PCR, polymerase chain reaction.

Plasma urea and creatinine are used to assess renal function. However, a significant amount of renal damage can occur before abnormal values are detected in the blood. The preferred option to assess renal function is the calculation of estimated glomerular filtration rate (eGFR) which closely reflects true GFR especially at the lower (clinically significant) end of the range (see Chapter 2). A full blood count may show anaemia (due to blood loss or impaired renal function). Other important blood results are shown in Fig. 8.11.

Haematuria

Blood in the urine can be:
- Microscopic: blood is visible only under a microscope or on dipstick analysis
- Macroscopic ('frank' haematuria): blood is visible with the naked eye (>5 red blood cells per high-power field).

The degree of haematuria does not always reflect the severity of the underlying disorder.

Causes

Causes of haematuria are:
- Renal causes: glomerular disease such as primary glomerulonephritis (e.g. IgA nephropathy), disorders secondary to systemic illness (e.g. vasculitis, systemic lupus erythematosus (SLE)), carcinoma (both renal and transitional cell), trauma, cystic disease, emboli
- Extrarenal causes: urinary tract infection (UTI)*, ureteral calculi*, prostatic hypertrophy*, carcinoma of the bladder*, renal stone*, trauma, urethritis, catheterization, post-cyclophosphamide
- Systemic causes: coagulation disorders, sickle-cell trait or disease
- Others: anticoagulant drugs.

(*Indicates the most common causes.)

Dipsticks detect haemoglobin (not red blood cells) and will give positive results if there is intravascular haemolysis, since haemoglobin is filtered freely by glomeruli (haemoglobinuria). This can occur physiologically, after heavy exercise, during pregnancy or with prosthetic heart valves. If haemolysis is severe (i.e. in haemolytic crisis), the urine can become red.

Other conditions can cause a red-brown discoloration of the urine that can be confused with haematuria (e.g. porphyria, myoglobinuria, ingestion of some foods (beetroot) or drugs (phenolphthalein)).

Diagnostic approach

Fig. 8.12 shows the common sites of lesions causing haematuria. The significance of urinalysis is summarized in Fig. 8.13. Transient causes of haematuria should first be excluded with a MSU culture. eGFR should be measured.

Macroscopic haematuria is investigated with MSU culture, urine cytology and urological imaging, e.g. ultrasound and intravenous urogram or CT urogram. Finally diagnostic flexible cystoscopy is performed.

Microscopic haematuria should be measured with dipstick tests. One + of blood or more on two dipstick tests or any symptoms requires further investigation. This would include eGFR, urine ACR and blood pressure. Then renal ultrasound would be performed if the patient was young or urological imaging and cystoscopy if old or had risk factors for urological malignancy.

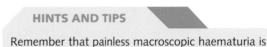

Proteinuria

Proteinuria is the presence of excess protein in the urine. It is usually assessed using a dipstick, which detects protein levels above 300 mg/L. 'Microalbuminuria' is the presence of excess urinary albumin but in amounts insufficient to cause a positive dipstick analysis. Proteinuria is best measured as the protein concentration on a 'spot' (early morning) urine sample corrected for urine creatinine concentration (protein to creatinine ratio or albumin to creatinine ratio). It may also be quantified on 24-h urine collections to give the amount excreted in 24 h but this is difficult to perform accurately and no longer routinely recommended. The amount of protein excreted can vary through the day and may increase with up-right posture (orthostatic proteinuria). Urine usually contains <20 mg/L of albumin and <200 mg/day of protein (exact values vary from laboratory to laboratory according to methods used to measure protein).

Proteinuria is seen in diabetic nephropathy. As well as being a risk factor for progressive chronic kidney disease (CKD), proteinuria is also associated with

Fig. 8.11 Blood test results and their significance.

	Indications	Scientific basis	Normal results	Abnormal results
Urea	Oliguria and anuria; dehydration; hypertension; diabetes mellitus; oedema; nausea and vomiting; loin pain	Crude indication of renal function	2.5–6.6 mmol/L	Increased in: Renal disease; high protein intake; fever; gastrointestinal haemorrhage
Creatinine	Same as above for urea	Reciprocal relationship with GFR–reflects renal function	60–120 µmol/L	Increased in all types of renal disease. N.B. GFR may fall by 50% before urea or creatinine go outside the reference range
Albumin	Oedema	Gives an assessment of severity of urinary protein losses in proteinuria	35–50 g/L	Hypoalbuminaemia Nephrotic syndrome Hyperalbuminaemia Dehydration
Sodium, potassium, anion gap	Confusion; lethargy; seizures; coma; arrhythmias; hypertension; hypotension; tachycardia/bradycardia; vomiting; diarrhoea; heavy sweating; diabetes mellitus; polyuria; polydipsia	Changes in the concentration of sodium, potassium and the anion gap are found in renal diseases; potassium is important in the function of excitable tissues and is important for survival	Na = 135–145 mmol/L K = 3.5–5.0 mmol/L anion gap = 8–16 mmol/L	Hypernatraemia Hyponatraemia Hyperkalaemia Hypokalaemia Increased anion gap in: Renal failure Ketoacidosis (diabetes mellitus) Hyperlactaemia (from shock) Anion ingestion
Arterial blood gases and pH (uses arterial blood)	Hypoperfusion; hyperventilation; Kussmaul's breathing in diabetic ketoacidosis; ingestion of acids; diarrhoea; vomiting	Oxygen concentration is important as it reflects tissue perfusion; an increase in CO_2 is lethal and poisonous to cells; pH is vital because most cells in the body work at an optimal pH and are very sensitive to changes in pH	pO_2 = 10.6–13.0 kPa pCO_2 = 4.7–6.0 kPa pH = 7.35–7.45	Acidosis commonly found in renal disease; compensated for by respiratory stimulation $\downarrow pCO_2$
Haemoglobin	CKD; haemorrhage	Haemoglobin levels are important as it carries oxygen to the tissues	Male 13.5–18.0 g/dL Female 11.5–16.0 g/dL	Decreased haemoglobin Chronic renal failure Blood loss Polycythaemia Renal tumours Renal cysts
ESR	Loin pain; symptoms of UTI; systemic disease		<15 mm/h	Increased in: Infection Renal cell carcinoma Retroperitoneal fibrosis Vasculitis
PSA	Any man aged >45 years with prostatism or UTI	The level of PSA increases with prostatic cancer and metastatic disease; used to monitor therapy success		Increased in: Prostatic carcinoma Silent recurrence of carcinoma Metastatic disease Small increase in prostatic hyperplasia
Urate	Kidney stones; patients with large tumour loads given chemotherapy; 'tumour lysis' syndrome → urate	Hyperuricaemia can cause urate deposition in renal tract	0.12–0.42mmol/L	Increased in: Gout Renal and urinary calculi
Calcium	Kidney stones; myeloma; metastatic disease	Hypercalcaemia causes calcium deposition in renal tract; hypercalcuria also causes urinary concentrating defects	2.0–2.6 mmol/L	Increased in: Renal and urinary calculi
eGFR	Monitoring known CKD, diabetes mellitus, hypertension, ACEi use	Estimates renal function from creatinine using MDRD formula, allowing for differences in muscle mass resulting from age, sex and race	>90 mL/min/1.73m²	Decreased in renal failure

UTI, urinary tract infection; GFR, glomerular filtration rate; PSA, prostate-specific antigen eGFR, estimated glomerular filtration rate; ESR, erythrocyte sedimentation rate; CKD, chronic kidney disease; ACEi, angiotensin-converting enxyme inhibitor. *MDRD, Modification of Diet in Renal Disease.

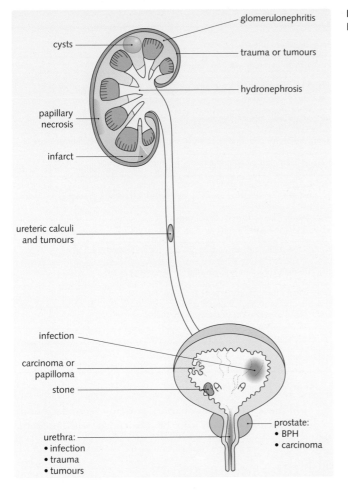

cysts

glomerulonephritis

trauma or tumours

hydronephrosis

papillary necrosis

infarct

ureteric calculi and tumours

infection

carcinoma or papilloma

stone

prostate:
• BPH
• carcinoma

urethra:
• infection
• trauma
• tumours

Fig. 8.12   Common sites of lesions causing haematuria. BPH, benign prostatic hypertrophy.

Fig. 8.13 Urine analysis – findings and their interpretations.

Findings	Possible diagnoses
Clots in urine	Carcinoma of the bladder or kidney clot colic is also a feature of IgA nephropathy
Albuminuria and haematuria red blood cell casts	Intrinsic renal disease glomerulonephritis – red cell casts are pathognomic of active glomerular bleeding (e.g. IgA, nephropathy, vasculitis)
Haematuria, pyuria and white blood cell casts	Renal tubulointerstitial disease –this is a non-specific diagnosis (i.e. pyelonephritis)
Dysmorphic red cells	Glomerular bleeding (i.e. glomerulonephritis)

increased cardiovascular risk in hypertension and ischaemic heart disease.

The causes of proteinuria are summarized, together with relevant investigations, in Fg. 8.14.

IMAGING AND OTHER INVESTIGATIONS

Imaging is a very useful investigation in renal disease when used in conjunction with other investigative techniques. Radiological imaging of the upper and lower urinary tract can be used to:

• Establish a diagnosis
• Assess the complications of impaired renal function
• Monitor the progression of disease
• Follow the response to treatment.

Clinical Note

• Imaging of the upper urinary tract includes KUB radiography, ultrasonography, CT, MRI and IVU
• The main form of imaging for the lower urinary tract is cystoscopy.

Fig. 8.14 Causes and investigation of proteinuria.

Cause	Investigation
Urinary tract infection	Mid-stream urine sample and culture
Diabetic nephropathy	Blood glucose levels (glucose tolerance test). Examination for other diabetic complications
Glomerulonephritis	Biopsy (for histological diagnosis). Blood pressure measurement
Nephrotic syndrome	Examination for oedema; urine ACR; serum albumin and cholesterol levels
Congestive cardiac failure	Clinical examination; blood pressure measurement
Hypertension	Regular blood pressure measurements
Myeloma	Full blood count Serum and urine protein electrophoresis Bone marrow biopsy
Amyloid	Congo red staining of tissue biopsy. Look for associated splenomegaly
Pregnancy	hCG (human chorionic gonadotrophin) pregnancy test
Pyrexia	Core temperature measurement at regular intervals
Exercise	Urine sample on waking to be repeated following exercise
Postural proteinuria (rare if >30 years old)	Urine sample on waking repeated at mid-day
Vaginal mucus contaminant	Repeat urine sample, with sterile technique

Plain radiography

Plain radiography of the kidney, ureters and bladder (KUB) is a simple, non-invasive test that can be used before specialized imaging. It is used to detect calcification in the kidney, such as renal and urinary tract stones – uric acid stones cannot be detected, but in general 90% of stones are radio-opaque (Figs 8.15 and 8.16). It also shows the size and position of the kidneys (this is unreliable), and any secondary bony deposits (such as can be associated with prostatic cancer).

Ultrasonography

Ultrasonography is a non-invasive technique that involves high-frequency sound waves. It can accurately assess the size, shape and position of the kidney, and

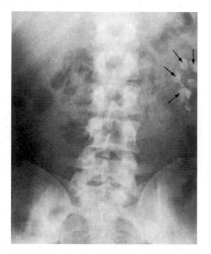

Fig. 8.15 Plain abdominal radiograph showing several calculi in the left kidney (arrows). (Courtesy of Mr RS Cole.)

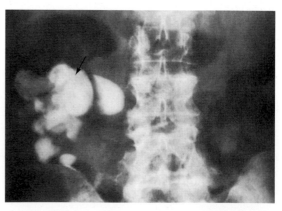

Fig. 8.16 This plain abdominal radiograph shows a large staghorn calculus (arrow) in the right kidney in a patient who presented with recurrent urinary tract infections. (From Williams G, Mallick NP, 1994. Color atlas of renal diseases, 2nd edn. Mosby Year Book.)

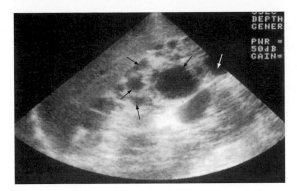

Fig. 8.17 Ultrasound scan showing the typical appearance of polycystic kidneys. There are multiple cysts (arrows) in the parenchyma. (From Lloyd-Davis RW et al, 1994. Color atlas of urology, 2nd edn. Mosby Year Book.)

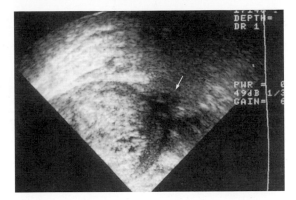

Fig. 8.19 A rectal ultrasound probe is used to define and stage carcinoma of the prostate. The arrow highlights an echo-poor area in the left peripheral zone of the prostate. This extends into the central part of the gland and beyond the capsule. (Courtesy of Dr D Rickards.)

can also distinguish solid masses and renal cysts (Figs 8.17 and 8.18). Dilatation of the pelvicalyceal system and upper ureters can also be detected – suggesting the presence of urinary tract obstruction. This is a major cause of reversible renal failure, and can be treated if detected early enough. Transrectal ultrasound (TRUS) can also assess prostate size and be used to guide a prostate biopsy (Fig. 8.19). Renal vein thrombosis can be detected with Doppler ultrasonography, and arterial Doppler studies can be used to identify renal artery stenosis. The specificity and sensitivity of ultrasound investigations are very operator-dependent.

Computed tomography

Computed tomography (CT) is a quick and non-invasive technique, which can be used with or without contrast. It is used to define renal and retroperitoneal masses and is ideal for locating and staging renal tumours (Fig. 8.20). It is also used to show polycystic kidney disease and has the advantage of also highlighting non-renal pathology. Modern techniques involving spiral CT can be used to visualize the anatomy of the renal arteries, renal vein and inferior vena cava, as well as retroperitoneal studies. Increasingly, CT without contrast is the investigation of choice to diagnose obstruction to the urinary tract or renal calculi (Fig. 8.21).

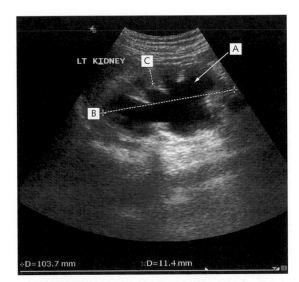

Fig. 8.18 Hydronephrosis of the left kidney demonstrated by ultrasonography. The echolucent (black) areas within the kidney are caused by dilated calyces (A). The bipolar length (B) of the kidney is normal and the cortical thickness (C) is well preserved, suggesting that prompt relief of the obstruction will allow good functional recovery.

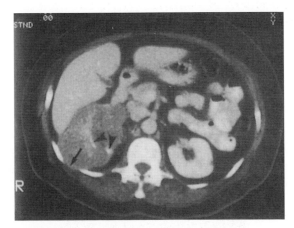

Fig. 8.20 CT scan highlighting a right renal cell carcinoma that extends through the intercostal space between ribs 11 and 12 (arrow) and medially along the renal vein. The high density (white) areas (arrows) indicate calcification. (From Williams G, Mallick NP, 1994. Color atlas of renal diseases, 2nd edn. Mosby Year Book.)

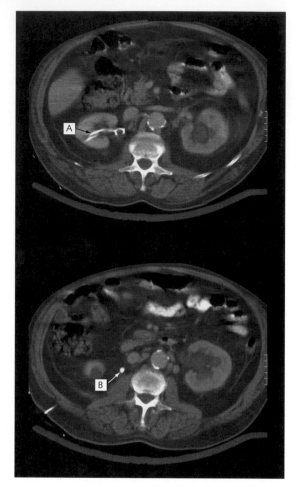

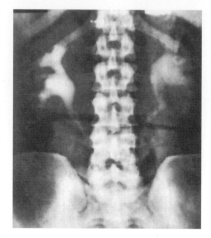

Fig. 8.22 An intravenous urogram showing bilateral hydronephrosis in response to bladder neck obstruction caused by dense granulation and fibrous tissue in a patient with schistosomiasis of the bladder. (From Williams G, Mallick NP, 1994. Color atlas of renal diseases, 2nd edn. Mosby Year Book.)

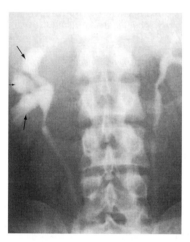

Fig. 8.21 An abdominal CT scan of a patient who presented with acute renal failure and bilateral loin pain. There is bilateral hydronephrosis secondary to bilateral ureteric stones. In the upper image a nephrostomy tube is seen in the right renal pelvis (A). The lower image demonstrates a dense opacity (calculus) lying in the ureter approximately at the level of L2 (B). Subsequent images demonstrated a similar opacity at L3 on the left.

Fig. 8.23 An intravenous urogram showing marked calyceal clubbing in the right kidney (arrows). There is gross dilatation of the calyces, which is pronounced in all poles of the kidney. These findings are the result of unilateral reflux of urine and chronic infection. (From Lloyd-Davis RW et al, 1994. Color atlas of urology, 2nd edn. Mosby Year Book.)

Intravenous urography and intravenous pyelography

Intravenous urography (IVU) and pyelography (IVP) involve serial radiographs taken after intravenous injection of radio-opaque contrast medium (Figs 8.22 and 8.23). Normal kidney function is required, and the patient must not be pregnant. An IVU can assess kidney size and shape as well as the anatomy and patency of the calyces, pelvis and ureters. It can also be used to localize fistulae and highlight filling defects in the bladder.

Investigations involving contrast involve the risks of allergy to the contrast medium and renal damage (especially if there is pre-existing chronic kidney disease). Allergy can range from mild (itching, nausea and vomiting) to severe life-threatening anaphylaxis. Previous reactions to contrast are a contraindication to its further use.

Renal arteriography

Conventional renal arteriography uses contrast medium to demonstrate the anatomy of the renal arteries. It is used to detect renal artery stenosis or aneurysms (Fig. 8.24). Therapeutic angioplasty may be performed

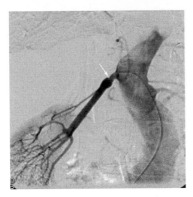

Fig. 8.24 Subtraction arteriogram of a right kidney. There is a single right renal artery with a significant stenosis at the ostium (arrow) with post-stenotic dilatation.

at the same time. It can also be used in the diagnosis of tumours, but this is becoming less common with the increasing use of CT. A catheter is introduced into the femoral artery, through which contrast is injected into the renal artery and a series of radiographs are taken.

Renal artery stenosis can also be detected using magnetic resonance imaging, avoiding the use of potentially nephrotoxic contrast (Fig. 8.25).

Micturating cystourethrography

Micturating cystourethrograms are used to demonstrate vesicoureteric reflux from the bladder to the ureters

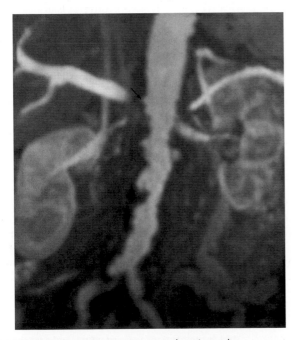

Fig. 8.25 Magnetic resonance renal angiography demonstrating a tight stenosis at the origin of the right renal artery (arrow). The irregularity of the abdominal aorta is due to marked atheroma.

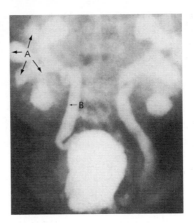

Fig. 8.26 A micturating cystourethrogram showing bilateral ureteric reflux. This patient has early calyceal clubbing (A) and ureteric dilatation (B). This is grade 3 reflux. (Courtesy of Mr RS Cole.)

during emptying of the bladder (Fig. 8.26). Reflux can be classified into three grades.

- Grade 1: contrast medium enters the ureter only
- Grade 2: contrast medium fills the pelvicalyceal system
- Grade 3: dilatation of the calyces and ureter.

This technique was used to investigate patients with recurrent urinary tract infections but has largely been replaced by other techniques because of concerns over ionizing radiation (especially in children).

Urodynamic studies

These are used to distinguish urge incontinence from genuine stress incontinence. They also detect bladder/detrusor muscle instability. The bladder is catheterized and a pressure probe is inserted to measure the bladder pressure. A rectal probe is also inserted to assess intra-abdominal pressure. The detrusor muscle pressure can be calculated by subtracting the bladder pressure from the intra-abdominal pressure. The bladder is then filled with water until the patient feels the urge to void. At this point the relative pressures are recorded. If the patient has stress incontinence, an increase in intra-abdominal pressure (e.g. coughing) leads to involuntary urine leakage, with no bladder/detrusor muscle contraction. If the patient has urge incontinence, the bladder/detrusor muscle contracts either spontaneously or with increased abdominal pressure, and the patient feels an overwhelming urge to urinate immediately (Fig. 8.27).

Retrograde pyelography

Retrograde pyelography is used to define the site of an obstruction (Fig. 8.28) or lesions within the ureter. It

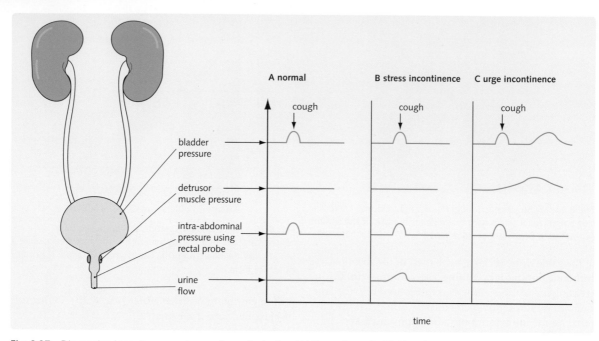

Fig. 8.27 Diagnosing incontinence using urodynamic studies. (A) Normal cough; (B) identifies stress incontinence, in which urine leakage is seen in response to raised intra-abdominal pressure; (C) shows urge incontinence, in which urine leakage is seen in response to detrusor muscle instability following a rise in intra-abdominal pressure.

does not require functioning kidneys. Under general anaesthesia a ureteric catheter is inserted into the ureter under cystoscopic guidance. Contrast medium is injected into the catheter to identify any lesions. It may be used therapeutically to help dislodge ureteric stones and coax them down the ureter.

Antegrade pyelography

This is used to define the site of obstruction in the upper urinary tract, i.e. mainly within the pelvicalyceal system.

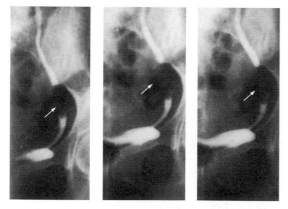

Fig. 8.28 Retrograde pyelogram showing a large filling defect in the left ureter (arrow) caused by a tumour. (From Lloyd-Davis RW et al, 1994. Color atlas of urology, 2nd edn. Mosby Year Book.)

Following percutaneous catheterization of a renal calyx contrast medium is injected as described above for retrograde pyelography Percutaneous catheterization of the pelvicalyceal system (nephrostomy) is also used therapeutically to relieve obstruction.

Magnetic resonance imaging

Magnetic resonance imaging (MRI) is an imaging technique that does not involve ionizing radiation – unlike CT. Instead, it relies on the measurement of the magnetic fields of atomic nuclei. It can differentiate cystic and solid renal masses and is useful for precise staging of tumours. However, MRI cannot be used in patients with pacemakers or other metallic implants. Magnetic resonance has now been developed to provide resolution sufficient to diagnose atheromatous renal artery stenosis (see Fig. 8.25). MR urography can also allow anatomical and functional evaluation of the urinary tract withouth the need for ionizing radiation or iodine-containing contrast agents.

Radionuclide scanning

Technetium-labelled dimercaptosuccinic acid (^{99m}Tc-DMSA) provides static images of the renal parenchyma. It highlights the localization, shape and function of each individual kidney, and highlights scarring as a result of reflux nephropathy (Fig. 8.29).

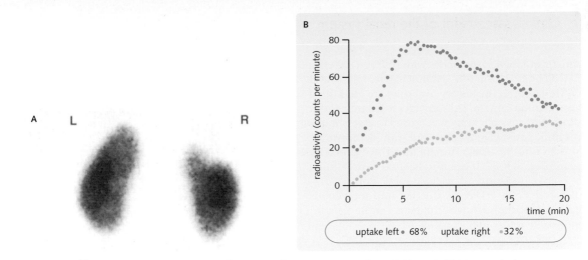

Fig. 8.29 (A) ^{99m}Tc-DMSA scan showing a right upper pole scar (courtesy of Dr TO Nunan). (B) The graph shows a diminished uptake of 36% for the right kidney, indicating a degree of loss of function correlating with the scar. (From Williams G, Mallick NP, 1994. Color atlas of renal diseases, 2nd edn. Mosby Year Book.)

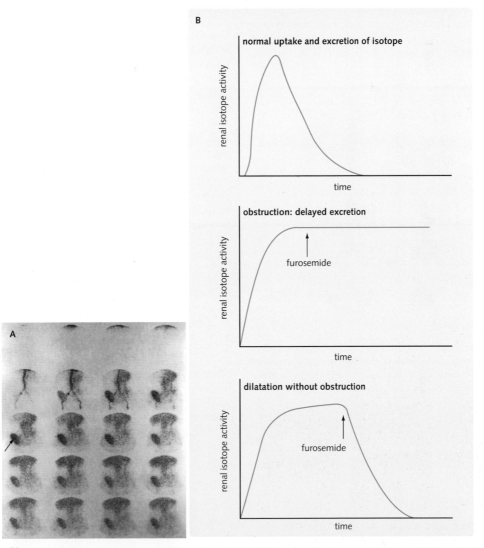

Fig. 8.30 (A)^{99m}Tc-DTPA diuretic renogram showing a transplanted kidney functioning normally (arrow). (From Catto GRD et al, 1994. Diagnostic picture tests in renal disease. TMIP.) (B) Diuretic isotopic renography showing tracings for normal, obstructed and dilated (without obstruction) upper urinary tract. Obstruction can be distinguished from dilatation by administering furosemide, which promotes excretion of the isotope in dilatation (without obstruction) but has no effect on excretion rates in obstruction. (From Johnson RJ, Feehally J, 2000. Comprehensive nephrology. Mosby Year Book.)

Technetium-labelled pentetic acid (^{99m}Tc-DTPA) is excreted by renal filtration and the changes in the level of ^{99m}Tc-DTPA in the kidney over time are quantified using a gamma camera. This provides a dynamic index of blood flow to each kidney. It is used to assess transplant function (Fig. 8.30A) and can demonstrate obstruction to the upper urinary tract (by diuresis renogram; Fig. 8.30B). It can also be used to determine the relative function of each kidney. Both ^{99m}Tc-DMSA and ^{99m}Tc-DTPA are injected into the venous circulation. Radionuclide techniques can be used to demonstrate reflux nephropathy.

Other imaging techniques

Other imaging techniques include scintigraphy. This may be used to investigate vesicoureteric reflux in place of conventional imaging techniques, avoiding exposure to large doses of X-rays. Scintigraphy can also demonstrate secondary deposits in the bone (Fig. 8.31).

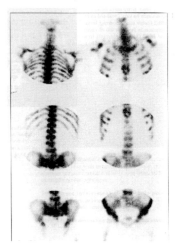

Fig. 8.31 This bone scintigram shows areas of increased activity in the ribs, sternum and pelvis (highlighted on the scan as dark 'hotspots'). This indicates multiple bone metastases in a patient with carcinoma of the prostate. (Courtesy of Dr TO Nunan.)

Cystoscopy

A rigid or flexible cystoscope is inserted through the urethra to inspect the interior surface of the lower urinary tract (bladder and urethra). This technique is very useful in the diagnosis and treatment of tumours in the bladder. It can also be used to identify stones and fistulae, to take a tissue biopsy and to assess prostatic disease.

Diagnostic cystoscopy can be carried out in the outpatient clinic, and involves a flexible cystoscope examination under local anaesthesia. Therapeutic cystoscopy may require a hospital admission and uses a rigid cystoscope, with the patient under general anaesthesia.

Renal biopsy

Renal biopsy is necessary to classify glomerulonephritis, which can influence the choice of therapy in patients with nephrotic syndrome and acute nephritis. It is also used in the diagnosis and assessment of systemic diseases that affect the kidneys, e.g. sarcoidosis and systemic lupus erythematosus. It can aid the investigation of unexplained acute kidney injury, proteinuria, and haematuria and is vital in the management of patients with renal transplants. A sample of the kidney tissue can be taken by inserting a biopsy needle into the kidney under ultrasound guidance, with the patient lying in the prone position. This is then examined under a microscope, using immunochemical staining to detect complement or immunoglobulins. Relative contraindications to renal biopsy include:

- A bleeding diathesis (absolute unless corrected)
- Single kidney (risk of loss)
- Obesity (technically difficult)
- Small kidneys (technically difficult)
- Pregnancy
- Renal failure (increased risk of bleeding).

The main complications are pain, bleeding (haematuria or perinephric haematoma) or infection (rare).

Single best answer questions (SBA)

Each question gives a list of five possible answers. Several may be true but pick the one that represents the best answer to the question.

Chapter 1 – Organization of the kidneys

1. Where do the renal arteries receive their blood supply from?
   a. The coeliac trunk
   b. The thoracic aorta
   c. The splenic artery
   d. The abdominal aorta
   e. The gonadal artery

2. What is the main anterior relation to the right kidney?
   a. Diaphragm
   b. Stomach
   c. Liver
   d. Pancreas
   e. Adrenal gland

3. The renal corpuscle consists of the glomerulus and Bowman's capsule. Where is it found in the kidney?
   a. The renal pelvis
   b. The hilum
   c. The medulla
   d. The cortex
   e. The papilla

4. Approximately how many nephrons are found in each kidney?
   a. 1 000 000
   b. 1000
   c. 10
   d. 100 000
   e. 100

5. What type of epithelium lines the proximal convoluted tubule?
   a. Simple cuboidal
   b. Stratified cuboidal
   c. Transitional
   d. Squamous
   e. Simple columnar

6. What connects the loop of Henle to the collecting duct?
   a. Proximal convoluted tubule
   b. Glomerulus
   c. Distal convoluted tubule
   d. Ureter
   e. Efferent arteriole

7. Which of the following is released by the kidney?
   a. Angiotensinogen
   b. Aldosterone
   c. Erythropoietin
   d. Anti-diuretic hormone
   e. Vitamin D

8. During development, if there was failure of cranial migration of the kidney what would this lead to?
   a. Horseshoe kidney
   b. Pelvic kidney
   c. Renal agensis
   d. Ureteric bud
   e. Metanephros

Chapter 2 – The glomerulus

9. The glomerular filtration barrier consists of fenestrated endothelium, basement membrane and what?
   a. Corpuscle
   b. Podocyte with filtration slits
   c. Mesangium
   d. Juxtaglomerular apparatus
   e. Filtrate

10. A patient is found to have a serum creatinine of 120 μmol/L. What can be calculated from this to form a better estimate of his kidney function?
    a. Modified MDRD equation to work out eGFR
    b. Clearance ratio
    c. Fractional excretion of creatinine
    d. Renal blood flow
    e. Muscle mass

11. In regulation of glomerular filtration rate, where is an increased filtration rate detected for tuboglomerular feedback?
    a. Macula densa
    b. Juxtaglomerular apparatus
    c. Efferent arteriole
    d. Afferent arteriole
    e. Bowman's capsule

12. A patient presents with severe ankle swelling worsening over the last week and proteinuria. Which of the following is the most likely diagnosis?
    a. Asymptomatic proteinuria
    b. Nephrotic syndrome
    c. Rapidly progressive glomerulonephritis
    d. Acute nephritic syndrome
    e. Chronic kidney disease

13. A 5-year-old boy has nephrotic syndrome. What is the most likely cause?
   a. Membranous glomerulonephropathy
   b. IgA glomerulonephritis
   c. Post-streptococcal glomerulonephritis
   d. Rapidly progressive glomerulonephritis
   e. Minimal change disease

14. Over the course of 2 days a patient develops oliguria, hypertension, fluid retention, uraemia, haematuria and proteinuria. Which of the following is the most likely diagnosis?
   a. Nephrotic syndrome
   b. Rapidly progressive glomerulonephritis
   c. Acute nephritic syndrome
   d. Chronic kidney disease
   e. Minimal change disease

15. A patient with glomerulonephritis develops haemoptysis. What could cause this?
   a. Goodpasture's syndrome
   b. Membranous glomerulonephropathy
   c. IgA glomerulonephritis
   d. Bacterial endocarditis
   e. Diabetes

16. What is an early indicator of glomerulosclerosis in a diabetic patient?

   a. Microscopic haematuria
   b. Microalbuminuria
   c. Anuria
   d. Macroscopic haematuria
   e. Uraemia

Chapter 3 – The tubules and interstitium

17. Name the process of transporting a substance against its concentration gradient, powered by moving a second substance down its own concentration gradient.
   a. Facilitated diffusion
   b. Secondary active transport
   c. Primary active transport
   d. Diffusion
   e. Osmosis

18. How do the convoluted tubules regulate body pH?
   a. Secretion of HCO_3^-
   b. Reabsorption of HCO_3^-
   c. Secretion of carbon dioxide
   d. Reabsorption of H^+
   e. Reabsorption of ammonia

19. A young diabetic is admitted with malaise and breathlessness. An Arterial blood gas analysis is performed with the following results: pH $=7.32$ (normal range 7.35–7.45), $pCO_2 = 3.5$ kPa

(4.7–6.0), $HCO_3^- = 14.2$ mmol/l (22–26), $pO_2 = 14.3$ kPa (>10). What pattern of acid–base disturbance is this?
   a. Metabolic acidosis partially compensated by hypoventilation
   b. Metabolic alkalosis
   c. Respiratory alkalosis partially compensated by the kidneys
   d. Respiratory acidosis
   e. Metabolic acidosis partially compensated by hyperventilation

20. A patient comes into A&E severely breathless. Her arterial blood gas analysis is as follows: pH $=7.48$, $pCO_2 = 3.5$ kPa, $HCO_3^- = 23$ mmol/L, $pO_2 = 14.0$ kPa. What pattern of acid–base disturbance is this?
   a. Metabolic alkalosis
   b. Respiratory alkalosis
   c. Respiratory acidosis
   d. Metabolic alkalosis partially compensated by hyperventilation
   e. Respiratory alkalosis compensated by the kidneys

21. What condition could cause the following arterial blood gas analysis result: pH $=7.34$, $pCO_2 = 6.8$ kPa, $HCO_3^- = 27$ mmol/L, $pO_2 = 10.0$ kPa?
   a. Vomiting
   b. Chronic obstructive pulmonary disease
   c. Pneumonia
   d. Pulmonary embolism
   e. Anxiety

22. How does parathyroid hormone affect the kidney's handling of phosphate?
   a. Decreases phosphate reabsorption in the proximal tubule.
   b. Increases phosphate secretion
   c. Increases phosphate reabsorption
   d. Decreases vitamin D activation
   e. Decreases phosphate secretion

23. What treatment of hyperkalaemia actually removes K^+ from the body?
   a. Calcium gluconate
   b. Insulin
   c. Salbutamol
   d. Sodium bicarbonate
   e. Calcium resonium

24. Which of the following would NOT cause tubulointerstitial nephritis?
   a. NSAIDs
   b. ACE inhibitors
   c. Gold
   d. Penicillin
   e. Rifampicin

25. A patient presents with flank pain, fever, and vomiting that all started 2 days ago. Her blood tests reveal a raised white cell count and raised

urea. Urinalysis showed the presence of protein, blood and nitrites. What is the diagnosis?
a. Kidney stones
b. Nephritic syndrome
c. Cystitis
d. Acute pyelonephritis
e. Acute tubular necrosis

26. What part of the loop of Henle is impermeable to water?
a. Thin descending limb
b. Thick ascending limb
c. Thin ascending limb
d. Thin and thick ascending limbs
e. All of it

27. What blood vessel is involved with countercurrent multiplication in the renal medulla?
a. Vasa recta
b. Interlobular artery
c. Efferent arteriole
d. Arcuate vein
e. Arcuate artery

28. Where is body fluid osmolality detected?
a. Carotid body
b. Carotid sinus
c. Kidney
d. Hypothalamus
e. Pituitary gland

29. How does ADH increase water reabsorption?
a. Tight junctions
b. Aquaporins
c. Na^+/K^+ ATPase
d. Decreases GFR
e. Release of renin

30. A patient has very high concentration of Na^+ in his urine and hyponatraemia. What problem involving antidiuretic hormone could cause this?
a. Nephrogenic diabetes insipidus
b. Neurogenic diabetes insipidus
c. Syndrome of inappropriate ADH secretion
d. Diabetes mellitus
e. Renal failure

31. A hyponatraemic patient has signs of dehydration and high urinary Na^+. What could cause this?
a. Vomiting
b. Congestive heart failure
c. Nephrotic syndrome
d. Sweating
e. Diuretics

32. A patient on the psychiatric ward is taking lithium. Why might he develop an abnormality in his serum osmolality?
a. Neurogenic diabetes insipidus
b. Nephrogenic diabetes insipidus

c. Diabetes mellitus
d. Hyperthyroidism
e. Vomiting

Chapter 4 – Body fluid volume

33. Which fluid compartment contains the greatest volume of water?
a. Extracellular fluid
b. Intracellular fluid
c. Transcellular fluid
d. Interstitial fluid
e. Blood plasma

34. Where in the nephron is most of the sodium reabsorbed?
a. Proximal tubule
b. Ascending loop of Henle
c. Descending loop of Henle
d. Distal convoluted tubule
e. Collecting duct

35. How does most sodium leave the lumen of the proximal convoluted tubule?
a. Na^+/K^+ ATPase
b. Diffusion
c. Facilitated diffusion coupled with other solutes (e.g. glucose)
d. Through tight junctions
e. Passes into loop of Henle

36. Which of the following is released by the kidney?
a. Antidiuretic hormone
b. Angiotensin II
c. Renin
d. Aldosterone
e. Angiotensinogen

37. Where is angiotensin I converted to angiotensin II?
a. Liver
b. Lungs
c. Kidney
d. Adrenal gland
e. Pancreas

38. What is the primary action of aldosterone?
a. Potassium reabsorption
b. Sodium reabsorption
c. Sodium secretion
d. Vasoconstriction
e. Vasodilation

39. What effect does sympathetic innervation of the kidney have?
a. Release of renin
b. Afferent arteriole constriction
c. Increased H^+ secretion
d. Decreases Na^+ reabsorption
e. Release of prostaglandins

40. What is the commonest cause of hypertension?
    a. Essential hypertension
    b. Atherosclerotic renal artery stenosis
    c. Fibromuscular dysplasia renal artery stenosis
    d. Chronic glomerulonephritis
    e. Chronic pyelonephritis

41. Which of the following is NOT a cause of secondary hypertension?
    a. Cushing's syndrome
    b. Conn's syndrome (primary hyperaldosteronism)
    c. Oestrogen
    d. Adrenal Insufficiency
    e. Phaeochromocytoma

42. What is a common side effect of ACE inhibitors?
    a. Taste disturbance
    b. Hypokalaemia
    c. Allergic reaction
    d. Fever
    e. Dry cough

43. What is the most powerful diuretic group used in the treatment of heart failure?
    a. Osmotic diuretics
    b. Loop diuretics
    c. Thiazide diuretics
    d. Potassium sparing diuretics
    e. Carbonic anhydrase inhibitors

44. Which diuretic might cause hypokalaemia?
    a. Osmotic diuretic
    b. Spironolactone
    c. Amiloride
    d. Thiazide
    e. Carbonic anhydrase inhibitor

45. What would be a logical treatment for Conn's syndrome (primary hyperaldosteronism)?
    a. Amiloride
    b. Loop diuretic
    c. ACE inhibitor
    d. Thiazide diuretic
    e. Spironolactone

Chapter 5 – The lower urinary tract

46. Which of the following is NOT lined by transitional epithelium (urothelium)?
    a. Middle third of the ureter
    b. Lower third of the ureter
    c. Bladder
    d. Prostatic urethra
    e. Membranous urethra

47. Other than its ability to stretch, what is an important attribute of transitional epithelium?
    a. Resistance to trauma
    b. Allows transport of solutes

    c. It is ciliated
    d. It is relatively impermeable to urine
    e. Resists infection

48. Which of the following is under voluntary control?
    a. Detrusor
    b. Internal urethral sphincter
    c. External urethral sphincter
    d. Urethra
    e. Trigone

49. A year after a patient sustains an injury to the thoracic spinal cord which of the following may describe their micturition?
    a. The bladder does not contract
    b. The bladder empties intermittently with no voluntary control
    c. The bladder is constantly contracted
    d. The internal urethral sphincter does not contract
    e. The internal urethral sphincter is always contracted

50. A patient on your ward has urinary incontinence. Whilst sitting, he suddenly gets the strong desire to urinate and immediately passes a large amount of urine. What type of incontinence is this?
    a. Stress incontinence
    b. Overflow incontinence
    c. Urge incontinence
    d. Functional incontinence
    e. Mixed incontinence

51. A patient with benign prostatic hypertrophy develops dribbling urinary incontinence. What would you call this?
    a. Urinary tract Infection
    b. Overflow incontinence
    c. Urge incontinence
    d. Functional incontinence
    e. Stress incontinence

52. What is the most common type of urinary calculi?
    a. Calcium phosphate
    b. Calcium oxalate
    c. Uric acid
    d. Cysteine
    e. Complex triple stones

53. A patient presents with flank pain and a renal stone 3 mm in diameter is seen on imaging. What is the appropriate treatment?
    a. Analgesia and oral fluids
    b. Analgesia and fluid restriction
    c. Endoscopic surgical removal
    d. Open surgery
    e. Extracorporeal lithotripsy

54. What are urgency, frequency, dysuria, lower abdominal pain and tenderness the classic symptoms of?
    a. Ureteritis
    b. Pyelonephritis
    c. Urethritis

d. Prostatitis
e. Cystitis

55. What is the common presentation of schistosomiasis?
a. Recurrent haematuria
b. Proteinuria
c. Hepatic failure
d. Nephrotic syndrome
e. Chronic kidney disease

56. How might you treat benign prostatic hypertrophy?
a. Dihydrotestosterone
b. β antagonist
c. β agonist
d. α antagonist
e. α agonist

57. Why is benign prostatic hypertrophy more likely to cause urinary obstruction than prostatic carcinoma?
a. Its growth is faster
b. It affects the transitional zone of the prostate
c. It is associated with calculi
d. It affects the peripheral zones of the prostate
e. It predisposes to infection

Chapter 6 – Neoplasia and cysts of the urinary system

58. A patient developed CKD caused by polycystic kidney disease as an adult. His wife is in good health and is pregnant. What are the odds that their child will develop polycystic kidney disease?
a. 0%
b. 12.5%
c. 25%
d. 50%
e. 100%

59. Why might you be worried about the patient with polycystic kidney disease who has a severe headache?
a. Uraemia
b. Meningitis
c. Migraine
d. Subarachnoid haemorrhage
e. Hypertension

60. What is the typical prognosis with polycystic kidney disease?
a. Steadily progressive CKD
b. Stepwise progression of CKD
c. No affect on renal function
d. Sudden deterioration of renal function
e. Associated with recurrent urinary tract infections

61. A patient who has been on dialysis for several years for diabetic nephropathy happens to have an ultrasound scan. This reveals several cysts within the kidney. What is this likely to be?

a. Adult polycystic kidney disease
b. Child polycystic kidney disease
c. Acquired cystic disease
d. Renal cell carcinoma
e. Medullary sponge kidney

62. What is a 1 cm solid lesion of the right kidney found incidentally on post morten most likely to represent?
a. Wilms' tumour
b. Metastasis
c. Renal cell carcinoma
d. Benign renal tumour
e. Polycystic kidney disease

63. What does the triad of frank haematuria, right sided flank pain and a mass in the right loin represent?
a. Renal fibroma
b. Renal cell carcinoma
c. Acute pyelonephritis
d. Splenic rupture
e. Ureteric calculi

64. At what age does Wilm's tumour most commonly occur?
a. 1–4 years
b. 10–14 years
c. 20–40 years
d. 40–60 years
e. >60 years

Chapter 7 – Acute kidney injury and chronic kidney disease

65. A patient on your ward is feeling lethargic and is passing very little urine. His blood results reveal a high serum creatinine and urea. His urine analysis reveals a low urine osmolality of 300 mOsm/kg. What could be causing this?
a. Congestive cardiac failure
b. Renal artery stenosis
c. Hypovolaemia causing prerenal failure
d. ACE inhibitors
e. Acute tubular necrosis

66. Screening for early kidney disease using albumin–creatinine ratio is most important in patients with which of the following diseases?
a. Alcoholics
b. Diabetic
c. Patients on NSAIDs
d. Congestive heart failure
e. Urethritis

67. A patient has an eGFR of 27 mL/min/1.73 m². What stage of CKD is she in?
a. 2
b. 3a
c. 3b
d. 4
e. 5

68. A patient with severe sepsis following a perforated appendix has developed AKI with hyperkalaemia and acidosis that are not corrected by medications. What would be the next appropriate management?

a. Continuous ambulatory peritoneal dialysis
b. Haemodialysis
c. Haemofiltration
d. Renal transplantation
e. Automated peritoneal dialysis

Chapter 8 – Clinical assessment of the renal system

69. Which of the following would not cause an enlarged kidney?

a. Diabetes
b. Polycystic kidney disease

c. Hypertension
d. Renal cell carcinoma
e. Renal metastasis

70. How might you differentiate left kidney enlargement from splenomegaly?

a. The spleen feels smooth
b. The kidney is dull to percussion
c. The kidney moves down with inspiration
d. The spleen has a notched border
e. The kidney is best felt bimanually

71. Why might you auscultate the abdomen of a patient with renal disease?

a. Tinkling bowel sounds
b. Renal bruit
c. Radiation of heart murmurs
d. Normal bowel sounds
e. Aortic bruit

Extended-matching questions (EMQs)

For each scenario described below choose the *single* most likely diagnosis from the list of options.

Each option may be used once, more than once or not at all.

1. Renal function

A. Loop of Henle
B. Atrial natriuretic peptide
C. Proximal tubule
D. Water
E. Juxtaglomerular apparatus
F. Distal tubule
G. Urea
H. Bowman's capsule
I. Protein
J. Calcium

Instruction: Match one of the items listed above to the descriptions below.

1. The site of production of renin.
2. In the glomerulus, the plasma is filtered through the capillary wall into this structure.
3. 70% of filtered Na^+ is reabsorbed here by an Na^+/K^+ ATPase pump on the basolateral membrane.
4. Antidiuretic hormone increases the permeability of the inner medullary collecting ducts to this substance.
5. One of the actions of this substance is to reduce Na^+ reabsorption by the tubule, thus increasing Na^+ and water excretion by the kidney.

2. Systemic and renal disease

A. Hyperosmotic dehydration
B. Glomerulonephritis
C. Essential hypertension
D. Diabetes mellitus
E. Renovascular hypertension
F. Hyposmotic dehydration
G. Urinary tract obstruction
H. Central diabetes insipidus
I. Oat cell carcinoma
J. Polydipsia
K. Nephrogenic diabetes insipidus

Instruction: Match one of the conditions listed above to the features given in the statements below.

1. Polyuria that responds to nasal application of antidiuretic hormone (ADH).
2. Decrease in extracellular compartment volume, increase in intracellular compartment volume.
3. Haematuria and proteinuria, oedema.
4. Hypertension associated with increased plasma renin concentration.
5. Hypertension of unknown cause.

3. Diseases of the tubules and interstitium

A. Toxic acute tubular necrosis
B. Amyloidosis
C. Polycystic kidney disease
D. Urate nephropathy
E. Urinary tract infection
F. Sickle-cell disease nephropathy
G. Chronic pyelonephritis
H. Drug-induced tubulointerstitial nephritis
I. Goodpasture's syndrome
J. Ischaemic acute tubular necrosis
K. Acute pyelonephritis

Instruction: Match one of the renal diseases listed above to the case scenarios described below.

1. A 26-year-old woman who is 26 weeks pregnant, presents with a 2-day history of dysuria and increased frequency of micturition. On inspection of the urine sample, you notice it is cloudy.
2. A 63-year-old man who has vesicoureteric reflux presents to the GP's surgery with a 3-day history of fever, general malaise and loin pain. He says he had also noticed that he suddenly needs to go to the toilet without warning.
3. A 28-year-old male dies from a motorcycle accident in which he lost a lot of blood following trauma to his abdomen. Histological examination of the kidneys reveals infiltration of inflammatory cells and tubular cells, flattened and vacuolated tubular cells and interstitial oedema.
4. A 33-year-old woman undergoing chemotherapy for leukaemia goes into AKI.

5. A 30-year-old woman is found to have severe hypertension. Her mother reports she had bouts of 'undiagnosed' fever as a young child and wet the bed until age 12 following which she has always had nocturia. Urinalysis reveals the presence of protein.

4. Signs in renal and urinary disease

A. Diabetic ketoacidosis
B. Bacterial endocarditis
C. Benign prostatic hyperplasia
D. Kidney transplant
E. Prostate carcinoma
F. Nephrotic syndrome
G. Hypertension
H. Carcinoma of the kidney
I. Stage 5 chronic kidney disease (CKD)
J. Renal osteodystrophy
K. Anaemia in CKD

Instruction: Match one of the renal diseases listed above to the clinical features given the statements below.

1. Large firm mass in the right iliac fossa with an overlying scar.
2. Splinter haemorrhages present on the nails.
3. Pale conjunctiva.
4. Facial oedema.
5. Prostate feels nodular on examination.

5. Disorders involving the kidneys

A. Ectopic kidney
B. Membranoproliferative glomerulonephritis
C. Loop diuretics
D. IgA nephropathy (Berger's disease)
E. Renal artery stenosis
F. Nephrotic syndrome
G. Hypoplasia
H. Thiazide diuretics
I. Renal cell carcinoma
J. Hepatorenal syndrome

Instruction: Match one of the items listed above to the statements below.

1. A congenital abnormality of the kidney that predisposes to infection and stone formation.

2. This is characterized by the presence of heavy proteinuria, hypoalbuminaemia and oedema, due to the glomerular capillary wall becoming excessively permeable to protein.
3. The most common primary glomerular disease, causing recurrent haematuria, and in some cases, end-stage renal failure.
4. A cause of secondary hypertension, due to poor renal perfusion and stimulation of renin secretion.
5. These diuretics inhibit the Na^+/Cl^- co-transporter in the early distal tubule. They help reduce peripheral vascular resistance, and so are used to manage hypertension.

6. Lower urinary tract abnormalities

A. Hydronephrosis
B. Hypertrophied bladder
C. Benign prostatic hypertrophy
D. *Escherichia coli*
E. Bladder diverticula
F. Hypotonic bladder
G. *Candida albicans*
H. Complete bifid ureters
I. Prostatitis
J. Hypospadias

Instruction: Match one of the lower urinary tract disorders listed above to the statements below.

1. The effect on the bladder if there is a lesion of afferent nerves from the bladder.
2. A ureteric abnormality predisposing to infection, due to urinary reflux from the bladder.
3. One of the most common pathogens causing cystitis.
4. A 65-year-old male patient presenting with difficulty in starting to urinate, a poor stream of urine, post-micturition dribbling, frequency and nocturia is likely to have this condition.
5. Obstruction at any point in the urinary tract causes increased pressure above the blockage. This is the term for the resultant dilatation of the renal pelvis and calyces.

7. Blood and urine abnormalities in renal disease

A. Incontinence
B. Hyperkalaemia
C. Urinary tract infection
D. Hyperuricaemia

E. Conn's syndrome

F. 100 mg/L

G. Hypernatraemia

H. 300 mg/L

I. Uraemia

J. Syndrome of inappropriate ADH secretion (SIADH)

Instruction: Match one of the blood and urine abnormalities that commonly occur in renal diseases to the statements below.

1. Uncontrolled diabetes, incorrect fluid replacement, primary aldosteronism and fluid loss without replacement are all causes of this imbalance.
2. A urine dipstick test can typically detect proteinuria, when the level of protein in the urine is greater than this value.
3. This can result following treatment of lymphoma, leukaemia and in psoriasis. It can also be induced by drugs, such as thiazide diuretics.
4. This is a cause of hypokalaemia (plasma $[K^+] < 3.5$ mmol/L) resulting from increased renal losses.
5. Risk factors include diabetes mellitus, impaired voiding, sexual intercourse, genitourinary malformations and impaired voiding due to obstruction.

8. Symptoms and signs in renal and urinary disease

A. Chronic kidney disease

B. Polycystic disease

C. Nephrotic syndrome

D. Benign nephrosclerosis

E. Ureteric obstruction

F. Abdominal bruit

G. Peritoneal dialysis

H. Bladder outflow obstruction

I. Haemodialysis

J. Nephritic syndrome

Instruction: Match one the conditions listed above to the statements below.

1. Microscopic haematuria, proteinuria and hypertension are typical features.
2. Causes pain which typically radiates from the flank to the groin and iliac fossa (loin to groin).
3. A patient presenting with dry, flaky, tanned-looking skin, scratch marks and bruises on his arms and abdomen.
4. May suggest renal artery stenosis.
5. A cause of irregular enlarged palpable kidneys.

9. Renal responses to systemic disorders

A. Afferent arterioles

B. β-blockers

C. NaCl and water retention

D. Metabolic alkalosis

E. Chronic pyelonephritis

F. Angiotensin-converting enzyme inhibitors

G. K^+ and water retention

H. Metabolic acidosis

I. Thiazide diuretics

J. Efferent arterioles

Instruction: Match one of the items listed above with the renal responses given below.

1. The kidney's response to hypoperfusion.
2. A renal cause of secondary hypertension.
3. In renal artery stenosis there is angiotensin II mediated vasoconstriction of these vessels to maintain glomerular capillary pressure.
4. Acute renal failure may be precipitated by giving this drug to patients with renal artery stenosis.
5. In hypovolaemic shock, the acid–base balance is disturbed, because Na^+ is retained, and is involved in the co-transport of H^+, K^+ and Cl^-. Cl^- is reabsorbed in equal quantities, but there is increased H^+ and K^+ secretion, resulting in this state.

Chapter 1 – Organization of the kidneys

1. d The abdominal aorta, at level L1
2. c The liver
3. d The cortex
4. a 1 000 000
5. a Simple cuboidal epithelium, with microvilli on the luminal surface to create a large surface area for absorption. They contain many mitochondria, reflecting the energy expenditure on active transport
6. c The distal convoluted tubule
7. c Erythropoietin, this hormone is produced by the kidney in response to hypoxia. The kidney does have a role in metabolizing vitamin D to its active form
8. b Pelvic kidney

Chapter 2 – The glomerulus

9. b Podocyte with filtration slits
10. a Modified MDRD equation to work out eGFR, this a patient's serum creatinine, sex, race and age to give an estimate of glomerular filtration rate. It is used clinically to classify stages of chronic kidney disease
11. a Macula densa, this is an area of cells in the distal convoluted tubule that detects the Na^+ and Cl^- concentration and communicates this to cells in the juxtaglomerular apparatus
12. b Nephrotic syndrome
13. e Minimal change disease, this is the most common cause of nephrotic syndrome in children, membranous GN is the most common cause in adults
14. c Acute nephritic syndrome
15. a Goodpasture's syndrome, autoantibodies to type IV collagen found in glomerular and alveolar basement membranes
16. b Microalbuminuria, the glomeruli start to leak protein. ACE inhibitors are an important treatment at this stage to slow progression of the disease

Chapter 3 – The tubules and interstitium

17. b Secondary active transport, this includes symport and antiport

18. b Reabsorption of HCO_3^-, 90% of bicarbonate reabsorption occurs in the proximal tubule
19. e The low pH is caused by metabolic acidosis, e.g. from diabetic ketoacidosis. The low pCO_2 and high pO_2 indicate hyperventilation which is an attempt to raise the pH of the blood
20. b Respiratory alkalosis, anxiety-related hyperventilation could cause this. As the HCO_3^- is normal there is no compensation by the kidney recognizable yet
21. b Chronic obstructive pulmonary disease. This is respiratory acidosis partially compensated by the kidneys raising the HCO_3^-. Pneumonia and pulmonary embolism would more traditionally cause type 1 respiratory failure, with hypoxia but less change in pCO_2
22. a Decreases phosphate reabsorption in the proximal tubule. PTH is released in response to low plasma calcium concentration. It also increases calcium reabsorption, increases bone resorption and increases vitamin D activation
23. e Calcium resonium, binds potassium ions in the gut, increasing the excretion from the body. All the other drugs listed protect the myocardium or redistribute the K^+ intracellularly
24. b ACE inhibitors, these predispose to prerenal acute kidney Injury by reducing the compensatory mechanisms for maintaining GFR but are unlikely to cause tubulointerstitial nephritis
25. d Acute pyelonephritis
26. d Thin and thick ascending limbs. These are impermeable to water but are permeable to ions and actively pump ions out, thus reducing the concentration of the filtrate
27. a Vasa recta – these are looped vessels that descend with the loop of Henle into the medulla
28. d Hypothalamus, this sends signals to release ADH and regulate thirst
29. b Aquaporins, these increase the permeability to water of the collecting ducts allowing water to be reabsorbed
30. c Syndrome of inappropriate ADH secretion
31. e Diuretics, the high urinary Na^+ indicates a renal loss
32. b Nephrogenic diabetes insipidus, this can be caused by lithium therapy, it is an inability of the kidney to react to ADH to concentrate the urine

Chapter 4 – Body fluid volume

33. b Intracellular fluid, comprises around 30 litres in a 70-kg male
34. a 70% of Na^+ that is filtered is reabsorbed here
35. c Facilitated diffusion coupled with other solutes (e.g. glucose), into the tubule cell. This is secondary active transport coupled with the Na^+/K^+ ATPase on the basolateral membrane
36. c Renin. ADH from posterior pituitary, angiotensinogen from the liver, angiotensin II formed from angiotensin I by ACE in the lungs, aldosterone from the adrenal gland
37. b This is by angiotensin converting enzyme (ACE) which is predominantly found in the lungs
38. b Sodium reabsorption, this raises the ECF volume. Aldosterone also increases the excretion of K^+ and H^+
39. a Release of renin, if barorecetors detect hypotension the resulting increased sympathetic tone stimulates the RAS system
40. a Essential hypertension, accounts for around 95% of hypertension
41. d Adrenal insufficiency, a deficiency of aldosterone and/or cortisol would result in hypotension
42. e Dry cough, caused by the inhibition of the breakdown of bradykinin. Taste disturbance, allergic reactions and fever are rarer side effects and ACEi cause hyperkalaemia, not hypokalaemia
43. b Loop diuretics
44. d Thiazide diuretics, e.g. bendroflumethiazide. Loop diuretics also cause hypokalaemia. Spironolactone and amiloride are potassium-sparing diuretics hence are liable to cause hyperkalaemia
45. e Spironolactone. It is an aldosterone receptor inhibitor. Conn's syndrome is the overproduction of aldosterone by the adrenal glands leading to fluid retention and hypertension

Chapter 5 – The lower urinary tract

46. e Membranous urethra. This is lined by stratified squamous epithelium
47. d It is relatively impermeable to urine
48. c External urethral sphincter
49. b The bladder empties intermittently with no voluntary control. The sacral reflexes are intact but there is no communication with the control centres in the cerebrum

50. c Urge incontinence. This is associated with detrusor instability
51. b Overflow incontinence
52. b Calcium oxalate
53. b Analgesia and encouragement of oral fluid intake. Stones smaller than 5 mm diameter usually pass. Surgery and Extracorporeal lithotripsy are options for larger, more troublesome stones
54. e Cystitis
55. a Recurrent haematuria
56. d α Antagonist, these relax the smooth muscle of the bladder neck. Another treatment option is Finasteride, a 5a-reductase inhibitor that prevents the conversion of testosterone to the more potent androgen dihydrotestosterone
57. b It affects the transitional zone of the prostate, the area surrounding the urethra, therefore is more likely to compress the urethra

Chapter 6 – Neoplasia and cysts of the urinary system

58. d 50%. Adult polycystic kidney disease is an autosomal dominant condition. The gene has a very high penetrance
59. d Subarachnoid haemorrhage. Adult PKD is associated with berry aneurisms. A berry aneurysm of a cerebral artery can rupture to form a dangerous subarachnoid haemorrhage, presenting with a thunderclap headache
60. a Steadily progressive CKD. Although the progression varies between patients the worsening of renal function tends to be steady and predictable
61. c Acquired cystic disease. After some time on dialysis patients develop this. The cysts can undergo malignant change
62. d Benign renal tumour, e.g. fibroma or cortical adenoma. These are a very common incidental finding
63. b Renal cell carcinoma, but not all will present with this triad
64. a 1–4 years old. It is the most common malignant renal tumour in children

Chapter 7 – Acute kidney injury and chronic kidney disease

65. e Acute tubular necrosis, the low urine osmolality indicates a problem of the tubules concentrating the urine, suggesting intrinsic-renal AKI. The other answers would all lead to prerenal AKI (with high urine osmolality) and if serious enough could also cause acute tubular necrosis

66. b Diabetics, screen annually with U&E and an early morning urine sample for albumin–creatinine ratio to show microalbuminuria. This early sign of damage can trigger stricter prevention of progression of CKD

67. d Stage 4

68. c Haemofiltration, this causes less cardiovascular strain than haemodialysis and is more suitable for haemodynamically unstable patients like this one.

Chapter 8 – Clinical assessment of the renal system

69. c Hypertension, most causes of CKD, including hypertension, result in small kidneys

70. d The spleen has a notched border. The other options are true but do not differentiate the spleen from the kidney

71. b Renal bruit, a sign of renal artery stenosis

EMQ answers

1. Renal function

1. E   Juxtaglomerular apparatus – the tunica media in the wall of the afferent arteriole contains an area of granular cells, which secrete renin.
2. H   Bowman's capsule – the capsule is lined by a single layer of podocytes, which rest on the basement membrane.
3. C   Proximal tubule – the luminal edge of each tubule is made up of millions of microvilli, forming a dense brush border that increases the surface area.
4. G   Urea – ADH also regulates the movement of water out of the collecting ducts in the loop of Henle.
5. B   Atrial natriuretic peptide – it is produced by cardiac atrial cells in response to an increase in ECF volume.

2. Systemic and renal disease

1. H   Central diabetes insipidus – a problem with ADH production, rather than ADH resistance.
2. F   Hyposmotic dehydration – more salt is lost than water, such as in adrenal insufficiency.
3. B   Glomerular nephritis – the inflammation of the glomerulus makes the glomerular barrier 'leaky' and interferes with its ability to stop red cells and proteins being filtered.
4. E   Renovascular hypertension – renin release leads to vasoconstriction through angiotensin II which raises blood pressure.
5. C   Essential hypertension – the most common type of hypertension.

3. Diseases of the tubules and interstitium

1. E   Urinary tract infection – common is pregnancy due to high levels of progesterone and smooth muscle relaxation.
2. K   Acute pyelonephritis – the ascending infection causes the systemic signs.
3. J   Ischaemic acute tubular necrosis – the blood loss following the trauma causes hypoperfusion and ischaemia.
4. D   Urate nephropathy – in tumour lysis syndrome the sudden break down of tumour cells releases large quantities of uric acid. This can lead to acute kidney injury.
5. G   Chronic pyelonephritis – infection (usually in early childhood) results in chronic scarring and can lead to hypertension and chronic renal failure. This is a T-cell-mediated inflammatory response.

4. Signs in renal and urinary disease

1. D   Kidney transplant – usually transplanted in this position, with its vessels anastomosed to the iliac vessels.
2. B   Bacterial endocarditis – this causes a systemic vasculitis.
3. K   Anaemia in CKD – there is no iron deficiency here, just a decrease in erythropoietin.
4. F   Nephrotic syndrome – the loss of protein in the urine corrupts the body's mechanism of drawing fluid back into the blood.
5. E   Prostate carcinoma – it is usually hard, irregular and nodular.

5. Disorders involving the kidneys

1. A   Ectopic kidney – the kidney does not ascend fully into the abdomen, so the ureters can be obstructed by neighbouring structures
2. F   Nephrotic syndrome – glomerular basement membrane damage and increase in pore size allows greater permeability to albumin.
3. D   IgA nephropathy – this typically affects young men after an upper respiratory tract infection. IgA deposition is seen in the mesangium.
4. E   Renal artery stenosis – there are two types; atherosclerosis, which is common; and fibromuscular dysplasia, which is rare.
5. H   Thiazide diuretics – renal side effects include hypokalaemic metabolic alkalosis, hyperglycaemia, hyperlipidaemia and hyperuricaemia.

6 Lower urinary tract abnormalities

1. F   Hypotonic bladder – lesion prevents reflex contraction of the bladder, so it becomes distended and thin walled.

2. H Complete bifid ureters – this results from early splitting of the ureteric bud or the development of two buds. One of the ureters inserts abnormally into the bladder allowing reflux of urine
3. D *Escherichia coli* – *Proteus* species and *Enterobacter* are other common pathogens. *Candida albicans* causes cystitis in patients on long-term antibiotics.
4. C Benign prostatic hypertrophy – enlargement of the prostate, which compresses the prostatic urethra and the periurethral glands swell, affecting the bladder
5. A Hydronephrosis – there is unilateral or bilateral dilation of the renal tract above the obstruction.

7. Blood and urine abnormalities in renal disease

1. G Hypernatraemia – serum sodium > 140 mmol/L. In the conditions listed there is an increase in solute to water ratio in body fluids, increasing serum osmolality.
2. H 300 mg/L – microalbuminaemia is the presence of excess urinary albumin but in amounts insufficient to cause a positive dipstick analysis.
3. D Hyperuricaemia – uric acid $= 480$ µmol/L for men, and $= 390$ µmol/L for women. It may cause gout.
4. E Conn's syndrome – hypokalaemia can also be caused by transcellular shift, and by extrarenal losses due to, among other things, diarrhoea and vomiting.
5. C Urinary tract infection – it can occur with or without leucocytes, caused by migration of bacteria up the urethra into the bladder, ureter and kidney.

8. Symptoms and signs in renal and urinary disease

1. J Nephritic syndrome – the signs and symptoms are decreased urine output, hypertension, oedema, haematuria, proteinuria and renal impairment.
2. E Ureteric obstruction – acute obstruction to the ureter typically causes pain with this distribution.
3. A Chronic renal failure – this can cause an increase in photosensitive pigment due to decreased clearance of porphyrins in the urine, and increased melanin secondary to increased melanocyte-stimulating hormone. Uraemia may also result in platelet dysfunction causing bruising.
4. F Abdominal bruit – this is the noise caused by turbulent blood flow through the narrowed arteries.
5. B Polycystic disease – multiple cysts develop in the kidneys from dilated tubules and Bowman's capsules.

9. Renal responses to systemic disorders

1. C NaCl and water retention – CCF leads to a fall in CO, causing renal hypoperfusion.
2. E Chronic pyelonephritis – Chronic glomerulonephritis and polycystic kidney disease are also causes.
3. J Efferent arterioles – constriction of the efferent arteriole by angiotensin maintains glomerular capillary pressure and glomerular filtration rate.
4. F Angiotensin-converting enzyme inhibitors – they are used to treat hypertension as they decrease the production of angiotensin II so decrease vasoconstriction.
5. D Metabolic alkalosis – this is also known as contraction alkalosis. Hypokalaemia also occurs in hypovolaemic shock.

Glossary

Acute kidney injury (AKI) A significant deterioration in renal function occurring over hours or days. Clinically, there may be no symptoms or signs, but oliguria (urine volume <400 mL/24 h) is common.

Agenesis A condition in which a part of the body (such as an organ or a tissue) does not completely develop or fails to develop at all.

Albumin A plasma protein synthesized by the liver, responsible for maintaining blood volume by its osmotic tendencies.

Anaplastic Characteristics of a cell (structure and orientation) that make it identifiable as a cancer cell and malignant.

Antidiuretic hormone (ADH) A hormone released from the posterior pituitary, which acts to increase water reabsorption from the collecting tubules.

Anuria No urine production.

Aquaporins Protein water channels, involved in the reabsorption of water in the collecting tubules.

Chronic kidney disease (CKD) The presence of structural and/or functional alterations within the kidney. It may (but doesn't always) lead to irreversible loss of renal function which is termed chronic renal failure.

Countercurrent multiplier The process by which the loop of Henle and the vasa recta system maintain a hypertonic medulla to concentrate urine.

Creatinine A waste product of protein metabolism. It is excreted by the kidneys predominantly as a result of glomerular filtration.

Davenport diagram A diagram showing acid–base disturbances and their compensatory mechanisms.

Diabetes insipidus Failure of ADH secretion or action; neurogenic or nephrogenic.

Dysplasia Abnormality of development, alteration in size, shape and organization of adult cells.

Erythropoiesis Process of erythrocyte production.

Glomerular filtration rate (GFR) The amount of filtrate that is produced from the blood flowing through the glomerulus per unit time.

Glycosuria The presence of glucose in the urine.

Gram's stain A stain for bacterial cells, used as a prime method of identification. Bacteria are divided into Gram negative, those bacteria which lose the stain, and Gram positive, those which retain the stain. These differences are based on variations in the structure of the cell walls of the different groups.

Haematocrit The percentage of red blood cells in total blood volume.

Haematuria The passage of blood in the urine. This may be seen by the naked eye (frank haematuria) or urine microscopy (microscopic haematuria).

Hydronephrosis Abnormal dilatation of a kidney; may occur secondary to acute ureteral obstruction (kidney stone).

Hydrostatic pressure The pressure of a fluid depending on arteriole blood pressure, resistance and venous blood pressure.

Intramural Being within the substance of the walls of an organ.

MDRD equation Equation used to calculate eGFR, which takes into account the serum creatinine level, age, sex and race of the patient.

Mesenchyme Embryonic tissue of mesodermal origin.

Nephrectomy The surgical removal of a kidney.

Oliguria Production of a diminished amount of urine in relation to the fluid intake (<400 mL/day).

Osmotic pressure The pressure of a fluid's osmotic effect due to the presence of plasma proteins and the imbalance of ions.

Osteodystrophy Defective bone formation.

Parenchyma The essential elements of an organ, used in anatomical nomenclature as a general term to designate the functional elements of an organ, as distinguished from its framework or stroma.

Percutaneous Performed through the skin.

Polycythaemia Increase in the haemoglobin content of the blood, either because of a reduction in plasma volume or an increase in red cell numbers.

Proteinuria The presence of protein in the urine. This may indicate damage to, or disease of, the kidneys.

Renin–angiotensin–aldosterone axis A molecular cascade stimulated in response to a falling extracellular fluid volume in order to maintain Na^+ balance.

Retroperitoneal Posterior to the peritoneum.

Sclerosis The development of fibrosis usually following inflammation (i.e. glomerulosclerosis).

SIADH Syndrome of inappropriate ADH secretion.

Tophi Pleural of tophus, a hard deposit of crystalline uric acid and its salts in the skin, cartilage or joints.

Uraemia The constellation of signs and symptoms that result from the accumulation of nitrogenous waste products.

Index

Note: Page numbers followed by *b* indicate boxes and *f* indicate figures.